MEDICAL APHORISMS

TREATISES 16–21

◆

THE MEDICAL WORKS OF MOSES MAIMONIDES

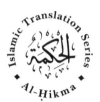

Maimonides

Medical Aphorisms
Treatises 16–21

كتاب الفصول في الطبّ

A parallel Arabic-English edition
edited, translated, and annotated by
Gerrit Bos

• • •

PART OF THE MEDICAL WORKS
OF MOSES MAIMONIDES

Brigham Young University Press ◆ *Provo, Utah*

Library of Congress Cataloging-in-Publication Data

Maimonides, Moses, 1135-1204, author.
  Medical aphorisms. Treatises 16-21 : a parallel Arabic-English edition / Maimonides ;
edited, translated, and annotated by Gerrit Bos. -- First edition.
        p. ; cm. -- (The medical works of Moses Maimonides)
  Parallel title: Kitab al-fusul fi al-tibb
  Includes bibliographical references and index.
  ISBN 978-0-8425-2863-4 (alk. paper)
  I. Bos, Gerrit, 1948- editor, translator. II. Maimonides, Moses,
1135-1204. Kitab al-fusul fi al-tibb. Treatises 16-21. III. Maimonides,
Moses, 1135-1204. Kitab al-fusul fi al-tibb. Treatises 16-21. English
IV. Middle Eastern Texts Initiative (Brigham Young University), issuing
body. V. Title. VI. Title: Kitab al-fusul fi al-tibb. VII. Series:
Maimonides, Moses, 1135-1204. Medical works of Moses Maimonides.
  [DNLM: 1. Medicine--Aphorisms and Proverbs. WZ 290]
  R733
  610--dc23   2015010268

Printed in the United States of America.

First Edition

Contents

◆ ◆ ◆

Kitāb al fuṣūl fī al-ṭibb (Medical Aphorisms)

◆ ◆ ◆

Sigla and Abbreviations

Arabic Manuscripts of Maimonides'
Medical Aphorisms (Kitāb al-fuṣul fī al-ṭibb)

B   Oxford, Bodleian, Uri 412, Poc. 319, cat. Neubauer 2113; fols. 1–123.

E   Escorial, Real Biblioteca de El Escorial 868, fols. 117–26 (numbered in reverse order).

G   Gotha, orient. 1937, fols. 6–273.

L   Leiden, Bibliotheek der Rijksuniversiteit 1344, Or. 128.1, fols. 1–140.

O   Oxford, Bodleian, Hunt. Donat 33, Uri 423, cat. Neubauer 2114; fols. 1–78.

S   Escorial, Real Biblioteca de El Escorial 869, fols. 176–1 (numbered in reverse order).

U   Oxford, Bodleian, Hunt. 356, Uri 426, cat. Neubauer 2115; fols. 1–107.

Arabic Manuscripts of Galenic Works

A   Ayasofya 3593, fols. 48a–51b. Galen, *Fī sū᾽ al-mizāj al-mukhtalif (De inaequali intemperie liber).* Forthcoming edition by Gerrit Bos, Michael R. McVaugh, and Joseph Shatzmiller.

Be   Berlin 6231, fols. 235b–269b. Epitome of Galen, *Al-adwiya al-muqābila li al-dawā (De antidotis).*

C   Cairo, *Ṭalᶜat ṭibb* 550. *Tafsīr Jālīnūs li-kitāb Buqrāṭ fī al-ahwiya wa-al-buldān.* Arabic translation of Galen, *In Hippocratis De aere aquis locis commentarius.* Forthcoming edition by G. Strohmaier.

H   Paris, Bibliothèque Nationale, arab. 2853. Galen, *Kitāb fī manāfiᶜ al-aᶜḍāᶜ (De usu partium)*. Arabic translation by Ḥubaysh, revised by Ḥunayn.

W   London, Wellcome Or. 14a. Galen, *Kitāb al-mawāḍiᶜ al-ālima (De locis affectis)*. Arabic translation by Ḥunayn.

Hebrew Translations

N   Paris, Bibliothèque nationale, héb. 1173, fols. 1–92. *Sefer ha-Peraḳim*. Translated by Nathan ha-Meᵓati.

Z   Munich, Bayerische Staatsbibliothek, hebr. 111, fols. 1–83. *Sefer ha-Peraḳim*. Translated by Zeraḥyah ben Isaac ben Sheᵓaltiel Ḥen.

Other

Bo   Maimonides. *Aphorismi secundam doctrinam Galeni*. Latin translation by Giovanni da Capua. Bologna 1489.

m   Maimonides. *Pirḳe Mosheh bi-refuᵓah*. Hebrew translation by Nathan ha-Meᵓati. Edited by Muntner, 1959.

r   Maimonides. *The Medical Aphorisms of Moses Maimonides*. English translation by Rosner, 1989.

A superscripted 1 after a siglum (e.g., **G¹**) indicates a note in the margin of that manuscript. A superscripted 2 indicates a note above the line.

◆ ◆ ◆

<>	supplied by editor and translator, in Arabic text
[ ]	supplied by translator, in English text
add.	added in
del.	deleted in or by
om.	omitted in
emend. Bos	emendation by Bos
(?)	doubtful reading
(!)	corrupt reading

Transliteration and Citation Style

Transliterations from Arabic and Hebrew follow the romanization tables established by the American Library Association and the Library of Congress *(ALA-LC Romanization Tables: Transliteration Schemes for Non-Roman Scripts*. Compiled and edited by Randall K. Barry. Washington, DC: Library of Congress, 1997; available online at www.loc.gov/catdir/cpso/roman.html).

Passages from *Medical Aphorisms* are referenced by treatise and section number.

Foreword

Brigham Young University and its Middle Eastern Texts Initiative are pleased to sponsor and publish the Medical Works of Moses Maimonides. The texts that appear in this series are among the cultural treasures of the world, representing as they do the medieval efflorescence of Arabic-Islamic civilization—a civilization in which works of impressive intellectual stature were composed not only by Muslims but also by Christians, Jews, and others in a quest for knowledge that transcended religious and ethnic boundaries. Together they not only preserved the best of Greek thought but enhanced it, added to it, and built upon it a corpus of scientific and philosophical understanding that is properly the inheritance of all the peoples of the world.

As an institution of the Church of Jesus Christ of Latter-day Saints, Brigham Young University is honored to collaborate with Gerrit Bos and other members of the academic community in bringing this series to fruition, making these texts available to many for the first time. In doing so, we at the Middle Eastern Texts Initiative hope to serve our fellow human beings of all creeds and cultures. We also follow the admonition of our own religious tradition, to "seek . . . out of the best books words of wisdom," believing, indeed, that "the glory of God is intelligence."

—Daniel C. Peterson
—D. Morgan Davis

Preface

This edition of Maimonides' *Medical Aphorisms,* treatises 16–21, is the fourth volume in a series of five that will cover all twenty-five treatises. In this volume, Maimonides explores women's diseases, the regimen of health in general, physical exercise, bathing, food and beverages and their consumption, and drugs.

In addition to the five volumes of text and translation, a sixth volume containing the medieval Hebrew translations by Nathan ha-Meᵓati and Zeraḥyah ben Isaac ben Sheᵓaltiel Ḥen and a seventh volume containing an extensive glossary of approximately five thousand terms from the Arabic text with their corresponding Hebrew and English translations are in preparation. Once completed, the glossary will be added to the others that have been put on the Internet to be consulted by the scholarly community (see www.uni-koeln.de/phil-fak/juda/forschung/forschungsprojekte/maimonides/glossare.htm).

This edition of the *Medical Aphorisms* is part of an ongoing project to critically edit Maimonides' medical works that have not been edited at all or have been edited in unreliable editions. The project started in 1995 at the University College London, with the support of the Wellcome Trust, and was continued at the University of Cologne with the support of the Deutsche Forschungsgemeinschaft. So far it has resulted in the publication of critical editions of Maimonides' *On Asthma* (2 vols.), *Medical Aphorisms* 1–21 (4 vols.), *On Poisons and the Protection against Lethal Drugs, On Hemorrhoids,* and the *On Rules regarding the Practical Part of the Medical Art.*

The series is published by the Middle Eastern Texts Initiative at Brigham Young University's Neal A. Maxwell Institute for Religious Scholarship. On this occasion I thank Professor Daniel C. Peterson, under whose direction this series was inaugurated, and his colleague,

Dr. D. Morgan Davis, for his continuing enthusiastic support and dedication to the project. Thanks are also due to Muḥammad S. Eissa, Angela C. Barrionuevo, Felix Hedderich, Sandra Thorne, Don L. Brugger, and Andrew Heiss for their diligent editing, proofreading, and typesetting. I also thank Professor Vivian Nutton for his help in correctly understanding and translating several Greek passages from the Galenic medical corpus. Finally, special thanks are due Dr. David Calabro for his careful review of plant names and taxonomies in this volume.

Introduction

This fourth volume of the critical edition of Moses Maimonides'[1] *Medical Aphorisms* covers treatises 16–21. The central subjects of these treatises are, respectively, women's diseases, the regimen of health in general, physical exercise, bathing, foods and beverages and their consumption, and drugs.

Treatises 17–20 aroused the special interest of the seventeenth-century Jewish Italian physician Jacob Zahalon. Zahalon found the aphorisms dealing with the subject of the regimen of health in general so valuable that—using a Latin version—he translated several of them into Hebrew and inserted them into his books *Morashah Kehillat Yaʿakov* and *Otsar ha-Ḥayyim* (first version) and into his commentary on Maimonides' *Hilkhot Deʿot*.[2] Treatise 19, on bathing, is quoted in the work *De balneis*, the most complete collection of early texts by Greek, Latin, and Arabic writers on balneology, edited by Tomaso Giunta and published in Venice in 1553.[3] Charting the history of bathing and containing precise descriptions of over two hundred spas, this work offers a unique sixteenth-century picture of what was then a very popular pastime, as balneotherapy was a fashionable means of treating medical conditions.

Most of the aphorisms found in this volume are based on the works of Galen, but Maimonides also quotes from other ancient and medieval physicians. An example of such a physician is Ibn Wāfid (eleventh century) from Toledo. He is Maimonides' primary source for a list of 265

---

1. For Maimonides' biographical and bibliographical data, see Bos's introductions to Maimonides, *On Asthma* (ed. and trans. Bos), xxiv–xxxiii; and Maimonides, *Medical Aphorisms* (ed. and trans. Bos), 1:xix–xxxii.

2. Cf. Zahalon, *Shemirat ha-beriʾut leha-Rambam*, 26–27.

3. Giunta, ed., *De balneis*; and see Friedenwald, *Jews and Medicine*, 1:203n31.

drugs to be taken internally and 20 drugs to be applied externally, which are commonly found in all places and which every physician should memorize.[4] Maimonides remarks that his decision to consult Ibn Wāfid's pharmacopoeia was based on the Toledan's being "known for his skill and for his correct quotations from Galen and others" (aphorism 21.67). While Ibn Wāfid was his major source, Maimonides adds that for some of the mineral drugs he relies upon Ibn Sīnā. Another source, consulted by Maimonides for the explanation of drug names in treatise 21, is Marwān ibn Janāh's *Kitāb al-Talkhīṣ*.[5] Maimonides' familiarity with this particular work is borne out by his statement in the *Glossary of Drug Names* that he bases himself on Abū al-Walīd ibn Janāh for the explanations of drug names.[6]

Sometimes Maimonides quotes from a medical work that has not survived in any other source, as, for instance, in aphorisms 16.1, 3, 9, 14–16, 20, 30, 35. These quotations derive from Galen's lost commentary on Hippocrates' *Diseases of Women* (the authenticity of this work is uncertain; it is mentioned by Ibn Abī Uṣaybiʿah but not by Ḥunayn ibn Isḥāq).[7] On another occasion, Maimonides quotes from a Pseudo-Galenic treatise that has been lost in the original Greek but survives in the Arabic tradition. This is the case with the following quotation, which has not lost any of its relevance, from Pseudo-Galen's *De somno et vigilia*:

> One should not neglect the movement of one's body as scholars do, who diligently study the entire night and day. The body and all its limbs should be moved evenly, and every limb should carry out its activity so that both the internal and external parts of the body receive benefit [therefrom]. *De somno et vigilia.* (aphorism 17.4)

What makes this quotation especially valuable is that it is also missing in the surviving Arabic translation and thus must have been part of

---

4. See aphorisms 21.68–87.
5. Ibn Janāh, *Kitāb al-Talkhīṣ* (ed. Bos, Käs, Lübke, and Mensching, forthcoming).
6. See Maimonides, *Sharḥ asmāʾ al-ʿuqqār* (ed. Meyerhof, 4, and introduction, p. xxvii); and *Glossary of Drug Names*, trans. Rosner, 4.
7. Ibn Abī Uṣaybiʿah, *ʿUyūn al-anbāʾ*, 149. Cf. Meyerhof, "Schriften Galens," 542 n. 56; Ullmann, "Zwei spätantike Kommentare," 245–62; and Bos, introduction to Maimonides, *Medical Aphorisms* (ed. and trans. Bos), 1:xix–xxxii.

an original longer treatise that has not been preserved in the Arabic translation.[8]

Sometimes Maimonides quotes from a medical treatise unknown from bibliographical literature, as is the case with the following aphorism derived from a commentary by a certain Asklepios on Hippocrates' treatise *On Fractures*:

> We should not use white hellebore [*Helleborus albus*] in our times because of the bad [physical condition] of the people. Their bodies are full of phlegm; the hellebore attracts it, and the patient suffers from strangulation. Instead, we should use agaric [*Fomes officinalis*] and the like. This was mentioned by Asklepios in his commentary on [Hippocrates'] book on [fractures] and their setting. (aphorism 21.33)

The name of this commentator has posed a bit of a mystery for scholars. Leclerc remarks that al-Rāzī, in his *Kitāb al-ḥāwī fī al-ṭibb*, quotes a commentator to Hippocrates' *On Fractures* named Senflious, and that the Latin translator has rendered this name Herilius or Sterilius. He adds that this could be read as Simplicius.[9] Steinschneider[10] notes that سينبليقيوس (Sinblikius) is indeed the first commentator on Hippocrates mentioned by Ibn al-Nadīm in his *Kitāb al-fihrist*[11] but adds that this name does not show up in the list of commentators in Littré.[12] Ullmann identifies سنبليقيوس, that is, the name of the commentator mentioned in al-Rāzī's *Kitāb al-ḥāwī fī al-ṭibb*,[13] as Simplikios and adds that he is otherwise unknown.[14] However, it seems more probable that the name of al-Rāzī's commentator is a corruption of اسقلبيوس (*'sqlbyws*)—Asklepios—and that he refers to the same Asklepios as Maimonides.[15]

---

8. Pseudo-Galen, *Über Schlaf und Wachsein* (ed. and trans. Nabielek, 34).

9. Leclerc, *Histoire de la médecine arabe*, 1:235, 267. Cf. Steinschneider, *Arabische Übersetzungen aus dem Griechischen*, 308.

10. Steinschneider, *Arabische Übersetzungen aus dem Griechischen*, 308.

11. Ibn al-Nadīm, *Kitāb al-fihrist*, 415.

12. Littré, introduction to Hippocrates, *Oeuvres complètes d'Hippocrate* (ed. and trans. Littré), 1:80–132.

13. Al-Rāzī, *Kitāb al-ḥāwī fī al-ṭibb*, 13:159; the name actually appearing in this book is سنقليوس.

14. Ullmann, *Medizin im Islam*, 31 n. 12.

15. For another quotation from this lost commentary, see Maimonides, *Medical Aphorisms* 15.63–64 (ed. and trans. Bos, 3:69) and the introduction by Bos, 3:xiii–xiv.

On another occasion, Maimonides quotes from a known treatise
bearing a title unknown from the bibliographical literature. This is the
case with his quotation from the Pseudo-Galenic treatise *De theriaca ad
Pamphilianum*, which is also the first to be documented in the Arabic
medical tradition.[16] Maimonides quotes this treatise under the title
"The Treatise on the Preparation of the Theriac" (*Maqāla fī ʿamal
al-tiryāq*). It is usually referred to as *Kitāb al-tiryāq ilā Bamfūliyānūs*.[17]

As I showed in the introduction to *Medical Aphorisms*, volume 1 (treatises 1–5), in many cases Maimonides does not just reproduce the
Galenic text but reformulates it through abbreviation or addition. The
following quotation from Galen's *De usis* is a nice illustration of the way
in which Maimonides deals with the Galenic text:

> In seeking health, a bad but regular diet of food and drink is more
> reliable, safer, and farther removed from danger than if a person sud-
> denly replaces his diet with something else that is better.[18] There are
> things which are by nature peculiar to some people and similar to
> their nature while other things are not peculiar to them and not sim-
> ilar to their nature.[19] *De usis*. (aphorism 17.23)

Maimonides selects and combines disparate elements from Galen's
lengthy discussion that he considers essential and uses the second part
to explain the first part. The following quotation is an example of how
Maimonides abbreviates Galen's discussion by omitting nonessential
elements:

> Just as wine is extremely harmful for children, so for the elderly it is
> extremely beneficial. The wine that is most salutary for them is warm
> and thin and has a bright reddish color. It is the one that Hippocrates
> calls "tawny." *De sanitate tuenda* 5. (aphorism 17.28)

Maimonides omits all of Galen's concrete examples of Greek and
Italian wines that have either one of these properties.

An example of an addition to the Galenic text can be found in aphorism 16.13, where Galen remarks: "In the case of inflammations of the
uterus, be careful not to perform a venesection from the arm, because
this hinders menstruation. Rather, cut the vein above the ankle, but

---

16. Aphorism 20.52.
17. Cf. Ullmann, *Medizin im Islam*, 49n52.
18. Galen, *De consuetudinibus* (ed. Schmutte, 6).
19. Galen, *De consuetudinibus* (ed. Schmutte, 16).

plan to do so three or four days before the time of the woman's menstruation," and Maimonides remarks in addition: "Then you may also apply cupping glasses to both ankles." And when in aphorism 17.5 Galen formulates two objectives of healthy living—replacement of wastes and elimination of residues—Maimonides adds that the first objective should be carried out in order to furnish the body "with something similar and suitable according to its temperament." Maimonides' additions sometimes assume the form of an explicit comment, introduced by "says Moses" (*qāla Mūsā*), as is the case in aphorism 16.4:

> Says Moses: The aforementioned causes [for the retention of the menstrual blood] mentioned by him only pertain to the organ when the menstrual blood is still present. He did not mention here those causes that are dependent on the blood, namely when its quantity greatly diminishes, for then blood is no longer present. Therefore, he speaks of the retention of the menstrual blood and not of its cessation.

Another adaptation of the Galenic text is when Maimonides turns a more specific statement by Galen into a more general one:

> Soft food is easier and faster to digest in the stomach, to turn into blood in the liver and the vessels, and to be absorbed into every single organ that is nourished by it. But harder food is more difficult [to digest] and more slow to undergo all [these processes]. *De alimentorum facultatibus* 3. (aphorism 20.6)

This quotation is an adaptation of Galen's comments about the flesh of oysters—that it is the softest of the testaceans, that it relaxes the stomach more but is less nourishing, and that testaceans with hard flesh are more difficult to digest and dissolve but are more nourishing.

As noted before, Maimonides was an independent and critical physician who tried to eradicate prejudices and dictated dogmas in medicine, even if their source was a physician as venerated as Galen.[20] This fourth volume also bears witness to this critical attitude. We have seen how he highly regards and praises the pharmaceutical compendium of Ibn Wāfid from Toledo. More negative, however, is his opinion about the pharmacopeia entitled *Kitāb al-murshid* (The guide), composed by the physician al-Tamīmī, who hailed from Jerusalem and moved to Egypt

---

20. Cf. Bos, "Medical Aphorisms: Towards a Critical Edition," 42–45.

in 970 to serve the vizier Yaʾqūb ibn Killis. About this work Maimonides
remarks:

> This man who was on the Temple Mount and whose name is
> al-Tamīmī and who composed a book on drugs and called it *Al-murshid*
> [The guide], allegedly had much experience. Although most of his
> statements are taken from others and although sometimes he wrongly
> understands the words of others, he still, in general, mentions many
> properties of various foods and medications, and therefore I decided
> to write down those that are good in my opinion, whether foods or
> medications. (aphorism 20.82)

Manuscripts of the
Kitāb al-fuṣūl fī al-ṭibb (Medical Aphorisms)

The work is known to be extant in the following manuscripts:

1. Gotha, orient. 1937 (**G**); fols. 6–273 (fol. 7 numbered twice); Naskh
script.[21] A considerable section of the text, from treatise 6.10 (beginning
at *al-mawt*) to treatise 7.16 (ending at *min amthāl*), is missing.[22] Another
section, aphorisms 20.30–33, seems to have been missing from the original version used by the scribe and was added by him at the end of the
treatise from another version.[23] According to the colophon on fol. 273a,
the scribe copied the text from a copy of the original redaction of the
work by Maimonides' nephew Abū al-Maʾālī (or Maʾānī) ibn Yūsuf ibn
ʿAbdallāh.[24] The scribe adds that he found a note in the text at hand in
which Abū al-Maʾālī remarks that, in the case of the first 24 *maqālāt*,
Maimonides would correct his autograph notes and that he, Abū

---

21. Pertsch, *Arabische Handschriften*, 3:477–78; and cf. Kahle, "Mosis
Maimonidis Aphorismum," 89–90.

22. Other sections missing are aphorisms 20.30–33 and 25.56–58.

23. See the following statement on fol. 231a: وجدت عند المقابلة في هذه المقالة زيادة على ما
في نسخة الأصل وهي (When collating this version with another one, I found an addition
in this treatise to that found in the original version, namely, . . .), and on fol. 94a:
وجدت هذه الزيادة في هذه المقالة عند المقابلة من نسخة غير الأصل (I found the following addition to
this treatise when collating [this version] with another non-original version).

24. See the remark by the scribe at the end of treatise 24 (fol. 239a):
"Something like the following was written at the end of this treatise: This is
what I found in the copy written by Abū [. . .]: I did not make a fair copy of this
treatise until after his death—may God have mercy with him—and [A]bū
al-Zakāt the physician wrote: Praise be to God, who is exalted."

al-Maʾālī, would then make a fair copy and correct it in Maimonides' presence; however, that the text of the twenty-fifth *maqāla* was copied by him in the beginning of the year AH 602 (August 1205 CE), after the death of Maimonides, so the latter had not been able to do the redaction.[25] Although it is generally agreed that this manuscript has preserved the best readings,[26] it should be noted that in some cases the text suffers from a certain carelessness by the scribe, resulting in mistakes and corruptions. Moreover, the language he employs is sometimes extremely vulgar and colloquial. Another characteristic of the text is that the central issue of many aphorisms is indicated in the margin, using terminology derived from the text itself.

2. Leiden, Bibliotheek der Rijksuniversiteit, 1344, Or. 128.1 (**L**); fols. 1–140; Maghribī script.[27] The manuscript ends on fol. 140b with the following colophon:

> This is the end of the treatise—praise be to God—and the completion of the Book of Aphorisms of the most perfect and unique scholar Mūsā ibn Maymūn ibn ʿUbaydallāh, the Israelite, from Córdoba—may God be pleased with him. The copying [of the text] was completed in the month of May of the year 1362, according to the calendar of al-Ṣufr, in the city of Ṭulayṭula—may God protect it—and it was written by Yūsuf ibn Isḥāq ibn Shabbathay, the Israelite.

The calendar of al-Ṣufr was common in Spain, especially among Christians, and started about thirty-eight years before the Christian calendar.[28] Accordingly, the manuscript was written in May 1324 in Toledo. More than any of the other manuscripts, the language of this one conforms to the rules of classical Arabic; the influence of vulgarization is thus far less pronounced than in the others. Just like **G,** it has many marginal catchwords.

---

25. See Pertsch, *Arabische Handschriften*, 3:477–78; Kahle, "Mosis Maimonidis Aphorismum," 90; Kaufmann, "Neveu de Maïmonide," 152–53; Meyerhof, "Medical Work," 276; Kraemer, "Six Unpublished Maimonides Letters," 2:79–80n93; Sirat, "Liste de manuscrits," 112; and Stern, ed. and trans., in Maimonides, *Treatise to a Prince*, 18.

26. Cf. Schacht and Meyerhof, "Maimonides against Galen," 59; and Rosner, introduction to Maimonides, *Medical Aphorisms* (trans. Rosner), xiv.

27. See Voorhoeve, *Handlist of Arabic Manuscripts*, 85.

28. Cf. Dozy, *Supplément aux dictionnaires arabes*, 1:836; and Kahle, "Mosis Maimonidis Aphorismorum," 90–91.

3. Paris, Bibliothèque nationale, héb. 1210 (**P**); 130 fols.; Judeo-Arabic; no date.[29] The manuscript only contains treatises 1–9 (the last one incomplete), part of treatise 24, and the major part of treatise 25. Also missing are aphorisms 8.42–59. According to the inscription on fol. 1b, the manuscript was once in the possession of Rabbi Meir ha-QNZ(?)Y. The text has been copied carefully, so there are only a few mistakes, but the top section has been so stained that the first lines are hard to read.

4. Escorial, Real Biblioteca de El Escorial 868 (**E**); fols. 117–26 (numbered in reverse order); Maghribī script.[30] According to the colophon, this text was copied in the city of Qalʿa (Alcalá) by Mūsā ibn Sūshān al-Yahudī in the year 1380 (read 1388), corresponding to the year 5149 since the creation. The text offers a close parallel to **L**, both having many otherwise unique readings in common, including whole paragraphs not appearing in any other manuscript, as, for instance, aphorism 3.52. Like **L**, it has several marginal catchwords, but they are not as many and they use a different terminology.

5. Escorial, Real Biblioteca de El Escorial 869 (**S**); fols. 176–1 (numbered in reverse order); Oriental script; no date.[31] The text is missing an important section between aphorisms 10.28 (from المستدل) and 21.72 (عنّاب) and finishes at aphorism 25.58. The text of this manuscript is closely related to **G**.

6. Oxford, Bodleian, Uri 412, Poc. 319, cat. Neubauer 2113 (**B**); fols. 1–123; Judeo-Arabic; Sephardic semicursive script.[32] According to the colophon, the text was copied by Makhluf ben Rabbi Shʾmuel he-Ḥazan DMNSY (from Mans?) and completed on the eleventh of Elul 5112 (1352 CE).[33] Numerous Hebrew translations derived from the Hebrew translation prepared by Nathan ha-Meʾati have been added to the text above the lines and in the margins. The text suffers from many

29. Zotenberg, ed., *Catalogues des manuscrits hébreux et samaritains*, 223; Vajda, *Index général des manuscrits arabes musulmans*, 345.

30. Cf. Derenbourg, comp., and Renaud, ed., *Médecine et histoire naturelle*, 74–75; and Cano Ledesma, *Manuscritos árabes de El Escorial*, 65 no. 33.

31. Derenbourg, comp., and Renaud, ed., *Médecine et histoire naturelle*, 76; Cano Ledesma, *Manuscritos árabes de El Escorial*, 65 no. 33.

32. Neubauer, *Hebrew Manuscripts in the Bodleian Library*, 721; and Beit-Arié, comp., and May, ed., *Supplement of Addenda and Corrigenda*, col. 392.

33. May, in Beit-Arié, comp., and May, ed., *Supplement of Addenda and Corrigenda*, col. 392, states that Steinschneider refers to a physician by the name of Makhluf of Marsala, Syracuse (Sicily).

omissions and corruptions but does provide some unique variant readings, as, for instance, aphorism 3.22: المركّب—a unique correct version according to Galen's τῆς συνθέτου σαρκὸς.[34]

7. Oxford, Bodleian, Hunt. Donat 33, Uri 423, cat. Neubauer 2114 (**O**); fols. 1–78; Sephardic semicursive script; ca. 1300(?).[35] The text begins with treatise 23, continues with the end of aphorism 6.90 to treatise 24 (which is incomplete, with large sections missing), and ends with treatise 12. The colophon found at the end of treatise 12 reads:

كملت المقالة التاسعة عشر وعدد فصواها ألف الحمد للّه على حسن ع>...> والسلام
على المألّفين من اللّه >...> تمّ الكتاب في سنت الف ط"ג لחרבن ב"ש تم

The flyleaf at the beginning reads:

הדה אלכתאב יסמא כתאב אלפצול לאן אנמזג׳ קול אטבא והו שרח אלמוג׳ז והו
כתאב יסמא אלדכיראת אלאטבא בג׳מעהון לגאלינוס ופצולהו ואבא קראט ופצ׳להו
צחא וקול אלחכים מוסא אלקורטבי ופצול אבן זהר ועדד ופצולהון אללף פצל פי
אלטב ואמראץ׳ אלבדן מן אלראס ללקדם פי עלם אלאבדאן מנלראס לחד אלאקדאם
ופצול באלאכואץ לעלאג׳ אל נאס

The flyleaf at the end by the same hand reads:

כתאב אלדי כאן ענתי פי מצר נאקלתו פי סאלופכי״ פי זמאן צלטן עצמן תריך
ע׳ה׳ע׳ס׳ סנת אלדי כונת פי אליגורנא מע דודור מורין ורחונא לאליגורנא קדנא
שהירין ורחות אנא ומעלמי לאנגלאתירא קדנא סני וג׳ינא עלא ויניזיא קדנא שהר
וג׳ינא לשיו פי סנת ה׳ ותלאתתמיי״ ותלאתין וכמס׳. תאריך

The text has a few catchwords, some in Judeo-Arabic and some in Arabic. The beginning and end have been falsified, and the original figures of the chapters have been altered. This manuscript is closely related to **E** and **L**, sharing many characteristic readings.

---

34. Galen, *De usu partium* 12.3 (ed. Helmreich, 2:188, line 4).
35. Neubauer, *Hebrew Manuscripts in the Bodleian Library*, 722; and Beit-Arié, comp., and May, ed., *Supplement of Addenda and Corrigenda*, col. 392.

8. Oxford, Bodleian, Hunt. 356, Uri 426, cat. Neubauer 2115 (**U**); fols.
1–107, Oriental semicursive script; late thirteenth century.[36] The manuscript itself provides us with two dates on fol. 106b: 1535 and a second
date that is hard to decipher—possibly the year 1500. The text runs
from aphorism 10.5 (at الضرورة) until aphorism 24.27 and has the following colophon:

תמת אלמקאלה י״״ה בעון מאלך אלדוניה אלחכים עלא אל ספלייה ואלעלאויה
וחאכים עלא עלאוייה ואל ספלייה צחיב אל דוניה אל מצ״ייא. שנת ה״ר״צ״ה

The text on the flyleaf at the beginning reads:

האדא לשמעון אלחכים אלמערוף באבן חנין אלראיס פי מדינת בגדאד
אלמערוף בל עלם פל טב כתאב כט אבי עזרא רחמהו אלה קד נקלו מן כתאב קדים

A second text on the same flyleaf reads:

האדא אלכתאב אלעזיז אלשריף לחביש אלתפליסי ומפראתו פל אדויה מתעלקה
באכואץ אלצחיחה ואלמעדין ועדד אלפצול סתמאיה וסתה וסבעון בעון אלחי אלחק
אלקיום קד אן כתאב פי מדינה באביל פי שנת ה׳ק׳ג׳ה׳. כתבתו(?) באיבירייא
ובאירחמן ארחם [. . .][37]

The text on the flyleaf at the end (fol. 107a) reads:

תמאת מקאלה חביש אלתפליסי אלמערוף אבן חבש אלחכים אלעריף אלזאהיר
אלמאהיר אלעריף באלתקים ואלתלטיף אלכביר אלחריף עדד מקאלתהו סתה מאיה
וסתה וסבעין פל אדויה ואלמפרדאת [. . .]. אלמקאלת ועדד אלפצול מגמוע גמיע
סימן תהעו בעון [. . .] רחמאן.[38]

Just as in the previous manuscript, the beginning and end have
been falsified. Similarly, the headings and figures of the chapters have
been altered.

36. Neubauer, *Hebrew Manuscripts in the Bodleian Library*, 722; and Beit-Arié,
comp., and May, ed., *Supplement of Addenda and Corrigenda*, col. 392.

37. [. . .] באיבירייא ובאירחמן ארחם: Missing in Neubauer, *Hebrew Manuscripts
in the Bodleian Library*, 722; and Beit-Arié, comp., and May, ed., *Supplement of
Addenda and Corrigenda*, col. 392.

38. Missing in Neubauer, *Hebrew Manuscripts in the Bodleian Library*, 722; and
Beit-Arié, comp., and May, ed., *Supplement of Addenda and Corrigenda*, col. 392.

9. Göttingen 99. This manuscript was copied by Antonius Deussingius in the year 1635 in Leiden from the manuscript there (**L**).[39]

10. Istanbul Velieddin 2525.[40]

For the edition of Maimonides' *Medical Aphorisms*, treatises 16–21, the following manuscripts have been consulted: Gotha 1937 (**G**), Leiden 1344 (**L**), Escorial 868 (**E**) and 869 (**S**, from 21.72 onwards), Oxford 2113 (**B**), 2114 (**O**), and 2115 (**U**). These manuscripts can be divided into two main groups, namely **GS** and **BELOU**. The edition is mainly based on **G**.

The decision to edit *Medical Aphorisms* in Arabic characters, rather than in Hebrew ones, has been inspired by Maimonides' own practice. Recent scholarship gives reason to assume that Maimonides usually composed a first draft of his medical works, intended for private use, in Arabic written in Hebrew characters, and that these works were subsequently transcribed into Arabic characters when intended for public use. Thus, Stern remarks that "all of Maimonides' medical works were naturally published in Arabic script, since otherwise they would have been of no use to the non-Jewish public," and adds that Maimonides first drafted the text in Hebrew script, because the Hebrew script was easier for him, and then had it transcribed into the Arabic script.[41] Stern's point of view has been endorsed by Hopkins, who remarks that although we have sporadic autograph examples of his Arabic handwriting, Maimonides always used the Hebrew script when writing privately.[42] Other scholars have expressed somewhat different opinions in this matter. Meyerhof remarks that Maimonides composed all of his medical writings in Arabic, probably using Arabic characters, since he had nothing to hide from the Muslims.[43] Blau suggests that when addressing a general public that included Muslims and Christians (as in the case of medical writings), Jewish authors might have used Arabic script; but when addressing a Jewish audience, they wrote in Hebrew characters.[44] Langermann remarks that it seems likely that many of Maimonides' medical writings

39. See Kahle, "Mosis Maimonidis Aphorismorum," 89.

40. See Ullmann, *Medizin im Islam*, 167 n. 4. I was unable to obtain photocopies of this manuscript.

41. Stern, ed. and trans., in Maimonides, *Treatise to a Prince*, 18. Cf. Blau, *Judaeo-Arabic*, 41n6.

42. Hopkins, "Languages of Maimonides," 90.

43. Meyerhof, "Medical Work," 272.

44. Blau, *Judaeo-Arabic*, 41. Cf. Baron, *Social and Religious History of the Jews*, 8:403n42.

were originally written in Arabic characters and that only afterward were these transcribed into Hebrew characters.[45]

For editing the Arabic text, which is written in Middle Arabic typical for this genre, I have adhered to the guidelines formulated by Oliver Kahl. Morphological and syntactic errors and even grievous offenses against the grammar of classical Arabic have been neither included in the apparatus nor changed or corrected at all. Orthographic peculiarities have not been included in the critical apparatus either. They have been either adjusted to the conventional spelling or left in their original forms, as the need for clarity dictated.[46]

As with volumes 1–3 of the *Medical Aphorisms*, this edition is supplemented by a list of faulty readings and translations selected from Muntner's edition[47] of Nathan ha-Me'ati's Hebrew translation[48] and from Rosner's English translation of that edition.[49] Muntner's edition is based on a corrupt manuscript—Paris, Bibliothèque nationale, hébr. 1173 (**N**)[50]—and therefore has many errors. Since Rosner's translation follows Muntner's edition, it suffers from many mistakes as well. The list also provides the versions of these particular readings by Zeraḥyah ben Isaac ben She'altiel Ḥen, derived from his translation of the *Medical Aphorisms* (**Z**).[51] I also note a few examples of faulty readings by Zeraḥyah and correct ones by Nathan. It is my hope that on the basis of this list and ideally on the basis of future critical editions of these translations,

---

45. Langermann, "Arabic Writings in Hebrew Manuscripts," 139.

46. See Kahl in Ibn Sahl, *Dispensatorium parvum* (ed. Kahl), 35–38.

47. Maimonides, *Pirḳe Mosheh bi-refu'ah* (ed. Muntner).

48. Nathan ha-Me'ati (from Cento) prepared this translation in Rome between 1279 and 1283. For his data see Vogelstein and Rieger, *Geschichte der Juden in Rom*, 1:398–400; Steinschneider, *Hebräische Übersetzungen des Mittelalters*, 766; and Freudenthal, "Sciences dans les communautés juives," 69–70; Bos, *Novel Medical and General Hebrew Terminology*, 2:21–27, 95–99.

49. Maimonides, *Medical Aphorisms* (trans. Rosner).

50. See Zotenberg, *Catalogues des manuscrits hébreux et samaritains*, 215.

51. For Zeraḥyah's versions I consulted the manuscript Munich, Bayerische Staatsbibliothek, hebr. 111 (**Z**). On Zeraḥyah, who was active as a translator in Rome and who prepared the translation of the *Medical Aphorisms* in 1279, see Vogelstein and Rieger, *Geschichte der Juden in Rom*, 1:271–75, 409–18; Ravitzky, "Mishnato shel Rabi Zeraḥyah," 69–75; Bos, ed., in Aristotle, *De Anima*, ch. 7: "Zeraḥyah's Technique of Translation"; Freudenthal, "Sciences dans les communautés juives," 67–69; Zonta, "Hebrew Translation of Hippocrates' *De superfoetatione*," 104–9; and Bos, *Novel Medical and General Hebrew Terminology*, 1:121–27.

it will be possible to provide critical evaluations of the translation activity of these two prominent medieval translators. With this goal in mind, a supplemental volume containing a comparative Arabic-Hebrew-English glossary of technical terms used in the *Medical Aphorisms* is being planned. The Hebrew terms will also be listed alphabetically in separate indexes with reference to the comparative glossary. Thus, the glossary and indexes may contribute to our knowledge of medieval Hebrew medical terminology. They may also be used to amplify dictionaries of the Hebrew language or, ideally, to create a dictionary devoted to this particular area. During the compilation of the glossary, it became increasingly clear that both Hebrew translations are based on an Arabic text represented by manuscripts **E** and **L**, since they share several unique readings. As explained in the first volume of *Medical Aphorisms*, Zerahyah's translation is characterized by many terms in Latin and Romance, and these will be registered in a separate index.

Last but not least, at the end of this volume I have also provided a list of addenda and corrigenda to the first three volumes, resulting from the preparation of the edition of the Hebrew translation by Zerahyah. The publishers have also included some corrections to the sigla found in the introduction to volume 2.

MEDICAL APHORISMS

TREATISES 16–21

◆

In the name of God,
the Merciful, the Compassionate.
O Lord, make [our task] easy.

The Sixteenth Treatise

Containing aphorisms concerning women

(1) The harm caused by the retention of menses is seldom evident in the first month. It becomes evident in the second month, though it is [still] somewhat imperceptible. But in the third and following months the afflictions [resulting from the retention] become severe. Menstrual blood that streams to the uterus in the first month can be contained by it, but when it becomes full, and consequently the blood that streams towards it does not find an [empty] place, [that blood] rises, goes back to its former place, and putrefies, and this results in those severe afflictions. *In Hippocratis De mulierum affectibus commentarius.*[1]

(2) Four or five days before menstruation the woman should adhere to a thinning diet and then be bled from her legs to stimulate the menstrual blood. Along with this, she should ingest remedies with hydromel,

بسم الله الرحمن الرحيم

رب يسّر

المقالة السادسة عشر

تشتمل على فصول تتعلّق بالنساء

(١) ليس يكاد يتبيّن ضرر احتباس الطمث في الشهر الأوّل ويبان في الشهر الثاني شيئا خفيا، وفي الثالث وما بعده تعظم البلايا لأنّ الذي ينصبّ منه في الشهر الأوّل تسعه الرحم و إذا امتلأت بما ينصبّ ولم يجد ما ينصبّ موضعا رجع إلى فوق فيعفن فتحدث منه البلايا العظيمة. في شرح أوجاع النساء.

(٢) قبل وقت الحيض بأربعة أيّام أو خمسة ينبغي أن تدبّر المرأة بتدبير ملطّف وحينئذ

تفصد الرجلين لتدرّ الطمث وعند ذلك تشرب الأدوية بماء العسل والفوذنج النهري والبستاني

---

١ بسم الله الرحمن الرحيم ربّ يسّر] om. BELOU || ٣ السادسة عشر] السابعة قال حبيس التفليسي U ||

٥ ليس] لا B | ويبان] ويتبيّن BEL يبين OU | الشهر] om. BELOU | شيئا] بيانا ELO تبينا BU ||

٦ البلايا] om. O || ٧ ما ينصب] om. G¹L || ١٠ وعند ذلك تشرب] وذلك بشرب BELO ||

water mint[2] [*Mentha aquatica*], and cultivated[3] mint. Stronger than these are savin [*Juniperus sabina*] and Cretan dittany [*Origanum dictamnus*], either in the form of a decoction prepared from one of these or its substance [only].[4] The best time to take these drugs that stimulate the [menstrual] blood is when the woman has left the bath and dried herself. Similarly, the ingestion of the *hiera*[5] at that time stimulates menstrual flow. *De venae sectione.*[6]

(3) A retention of the menstrual blood results from the weakness of the vessels and the uterus so that they cannot attract it, or because of an obstruction there, or because of a contraction of the uterus. *In Hippocratis De mulierum affectibus commentarius.*[7]

(4) Says Moses: The aforementioned causes [for the retention of the menstrual blood] mentioned by him only pertain to the organ[8] when the menstrual blood is still present. He did not mention[9] here those causes that are dependent on the blood, namely when its quantity greatly diminishes, for then blood is no longer present. Therefore, he speaks of the retention of the menstrual blood and not of its cessation.[10]

(5) Retention of the menses is usually followed by some or all of the [possible] bad afflictions—namely, heaviness[11] of the body; loss of appetite; shivering; pain in the loins, neck, forehead, head, or roots[12] of the eyes; ardent fevers; a dark,[13] reddish urine; flow[14] of milk from the breasts. When the retention of the menses lasts for a long time, a swelling may occur in[15] the hollow of the groin. But those women who have a normal menstruation do not suffer from any of these afflictions. *De locis affectis* 6.[16]

(6) When the evacuation of menstrual blood becomes excessive, it is followed by a bad[17] complexion, swelling of the feet and the whole body, and poor digestion. *De locis affectis* 6.[18]

وأقوى من ذلك الأبهل والمشكطرامشيغ إمّا طبيخ أحدها أو جرمه. وأفضل أوقات أخذ هذه الأدوية المدرّة للدم عند الخروج من الحمّام والمرأة بعد تتنشّف. وكذلك شرب الإيارج في هذا الوقت يدرّ الطمث. في مقالته في الفصد.

(٣) احتباس دم الطمث إمّا من قِبَل ضعف العروق والرحم عن اجتذابه، أو من قِبَل سدّة هناك أو من قِبَل انضمام الرحم. في شرحه لأوجاع النساء. ٥

(٤) قال موسى: هذه الأسباب التي ذكرها هي من قبل الآلة فقط ويكون دم الطمث موجودا. ولم يذكر هنا الأسباب المتعلّقة بالدم أعني كمّية الدم إذا قلّت جدّا لأنّ دم الطمث حينئذ غير موجود ولذلك قال احتباس دم الطمث ولم يقل انقطاع الطمث.

(٥) احتباس الطمث تتبعه على الأمر الأكثر أعراض رديئة، إمّا كلّها أو بعضها، وهي ثقل البدن وانقطاع الشهوة واقشعرار ووجع القطَن أو العنق أو اليافوخ أو الرأس أو أصل العينين، وحمّيات محرقة وبول مختلط اللون من سواد وحمرة، ودرور لبن من الثديين. وإن طال احتباس الطمث فربّما ظهر غلظ في الموضع الخالي من الحالب. ومن كان من النساء يجري أمر الطمث منهن المجرى المحمود فليس لها يعرض من هذا شيء. سادسة التعرّف. ١٠

(٦) إذا أفرط استفراغ دم الطمث تبع ذلك رداءة اللون وتهيّج القدمين وجميع البدن ورداءة الاستمراء. سادسة التعرّف. ١٥

---

٢ بعد] أن add. B || ٧ ولم يذكر هنا] ولم يقصده هنا BELOU || ١١ وبول مختلط اللون من سواد وحمرة] om. G ١٢ || ومن] وما ELO || ١٤ إذا ... سادسة التعرّف] om. B

(7) Sometimes women suffer from the illness[19] called *nazf* [female flux] whereby the whole body is purged. This mostly occurs to those women whose bodies are soft and phlegmatic [in constitution]. The discharge [from the body] through this flux sometimes consists of a reddish serum and at other times of a watery or yellowish serum. But if you observe that the blood is like the blood of venesection, investigate it carefully to determine if it comes from an erosion. Most often, such an erosion occurs at the neck of the uterus. *De locis affectis* 6.[20]

(8) Just as there are men whose nature tends towards that of a woman and whose bodies are tender and soft, similar to [the body] of a woman, so too there are women whose bodies are dry and hard, similar to the nature of [the body of] a man. If the nature of a woman tends towards the nature of a man, there is nothing with which she can be treated to strengthen and stimulate her menstrual flow. *In Hippocratis Epidemiarum librum* 6 *commentaria* 8,[21] specifically the last part of the book.

(9) Superfluities accumulate in the bodies of women because of their state of rest, calm, and lack of exertion. Nature expels these superfluities to the vessels that are connected to the uterus; they accumulate there, for the uterus has the strength to attract these superfluities. *In Hippocratis De mulierum affectibus commentarius.*[22]

(10) All the pulsatile and nonpulsatile vessels in the entire body of both male and female are the same, not only in number but also in structure, form, and location. However, [male and female] are different in their reproductive organs. [Yet] it is clear from anatomy that the reproductive parts of the male and female correspond to each other and resemble each other, though in the male they protrude whereas in the female they are internal. [This is true] to such a degree that if the female [reproductive] organs were reversed so that their internal side would be external, the uterus would, as it were, become the scrotum, and the testicles,[23] which are on the sides of the uterus, would be located inside this pouch, and the neck of the uterus would correspond to the penis. *De semine* 2.[24]

(٧) قد يعرض للنساء العلّة المعروفة بالنزف عند ما ينقّى بذلك البدن كلّه. وأكثر ما يكون ذلك للنساء اللّينات الأبدان البلغميات. والشيء الذي يستفرغ بالنزف في بعض الأوقات يكون صديدا أحمر وفي بعض الأوقات صديدا مائيا أو يضرب إلى الصفرة. وأمّا إن رأيته مثل دم الفصاد فتفقّد إيّاك أن يكون من تأكّل، وأكثر ما يعرض التأكّل في عنق الرحم. سادسة التعرّف.

٥

(٨) كما أنّ من الرجال من مال طبعه إلى طبع النساء ويكون جسمه ناعما ليّنا شبيها ببدن المرأة كذلك قد يوجد في النساء من بدنها جافّ صلب شبيه بطبيعة الرجل. فكلّ امرأة تنقل طبعها إلى طبع الرجال فليس شيء من العلاج يقوّي على تحريك طمثها. في الثامنة من شرحه لسادسة أبيديميا وهي آخر الكتاب.

(٩) الفضول تجتمع في أبدان النساء من قبل سكونهنّ ودعتهنّ وتركهنّ التعب وهذه الفضول تدفعها الطبيعة إلى العروق التي تتّصل بالرحم وتجتمع هناك وللرحم قوة جذّابة لهذه الفضول. في شرحه لأوجاع النساء.

١٠

(١٠) جميع الشريانات والعروق في جميع البدن من الذكور والإناث معا على مثال واحد ليس في عددها فقط لكنّ في خلقتها وهيئتها ووضعها. وإنّما يختلفان بآلات التناسل، ويتبيّن في التشريح أنّ أعضاء التناسل في الذكور والإناث نظائر متشبّهة. وإنّما هي في الذكور بارزة وهي في الإناث باطنة حتّى لو انقلبت آلات الأنثى حتّى تصير صفحتها الداخلة خارجة لصار الرحم كأنّه كيس الأنثيين والأنثيان التي بجانبي الرحم تصير داخل ذلك الكيس ويصير عنق الرحم نظير القضيب. في الثانية من كتاب المنّي.

١٥

---

٣ يكون] om. BELOU || ٨ الثامنة] خامسة LO || ٩ أبيديميا] أفيديميا ELO || ١١ جذّابة] جاذبة BELOU || ١٦ صفحتها] ELO صفاتها صفيحتها B صفاته U || ١٧ بجانبي] بجنب ELO بجنبي BU | الرحم . . . عنق] om. G | تصير] يصيران ELO

(11) If too much [blood] is evacuated from the uterus all at once, apply cupping glasses next to the breasts and it will stop rapidly.[25] Similarly, place cupping glasses on the two groins and thighs of a woman whose uterus is drawn and raised upwards or is inclined side-wards.[26] Place something with an extremely repulsive smell near her nostrils and[27] sweet-smelling medicines with slackening and heating properties near her uterus. *Ad Glauconem [de medendi methodo]* 1.[28]

(12) Generally apply cupping glasses to the pudenda and groins if you want to promote and stimulate the [flow of] the menstrual blood. *De methodo [medendi]* 13.[29]

(13) In the case of inflammations of the uterus, be careful not to perform a venesection from the arm, because this hinders menstrua-tion. Rather, cut the vein above the ankle, but plan to do so three or four days before the time of the woman's menstruation. Then[30] you may also apply cupping glasses to both ankles. *De venae sectione.*[31]

(14) When a woman has a normal menstruation and performs light work, she does not desire sexual intercourse because her body is free from those superfluities that tickle and stimulate the uterus to seek sexual intercourse. *In Hippocratis De mulierum affectibus commentarius.*[32]

(15) When the flow of menstrual blood is excessive, the nerves and muscles on the spinal column stretch because of dryness, and this causes pain. Sometimes the uterus ascends when it suffers from spasms caused by the dryness resulting from excessive menstrual bleeding. With the stretching of the uterus, the diaphragm and the viscera also stretch and then [hysterical] suffocation develops. *In Hippocratis De muli-erum affectibus commentarius.*[33]

(16) Hysterical suffocation occurs if the menses are retained and if the uterus and the vessels that lead to the uterus and its ligaments are filled [with superfluous matter] and stretch, causing the uterus to stretch upwards and press on the diaphragm. Respiration then becomes difficult, and sometimes pressure on the stomach or on the organs lying on the spinal column causes severe pain. *In Hippocratis De mulierum affec-tibus commentarius.*[34]

(١١) متى كان من الرحم استفراغ كثير دفعة فوضعت المحاجم عند الثديين سكنت ذلك في أسرع الأوقات. وكذلك تضع المحاجم على الأربيتين والفخذين في المرأة التي قد تقلّص منها الرحم واستقلّ شاهقا أو مال إلى أحد الجانبين. ويدنى من منخريها ما له رائحة كريهة في غاية الكراهة ومن الرحم أدوية طيّبة الرائحة ومن شأنها أن ترخي وتسخن. في الأوّل من أغلوقن.

(١٢) كثيرا ما تعلق على العانة والحالبين محاجم عند ما تريد أن تحرّك دم الحيض وتستدعيه. ثالثة عشر الحيلة.

(١٣) احذر فصد العرق من اليد في أورام الرحم لأنّه يعيق الطمث. بل تفصد فوق الكعب وتتوخّى أن تفعل ذلك قبل وقت حيض المرأة بثلاثة أيّام أو أربعة. وحينئذ أيضا تعلق المحاجم على الكعبين. في مقالته في الفصد.

(١٤) من كان طمثها على اعتداله وهي تستعمل التعب قليلا فهي لا تشتاق إلى الباه لأنّ بدنها ينقى من الفضول التي تدغدغ الرحم وتهيجه لطلب الباه. في شرحه لأوجاع النساء.

(١٥) إن أفرط النزف تمدّد العصب والعضلات التي على الصلب من اليبس فيحدث وجعا وقد تتشنّج الرحم من اليبس العارض من كثرة النزف وتصعد إلى فوق ويتمدّد بتمدّدها الحجاب والأحشاء فيحدث الاختناق. شرح أوجاع النساء.

(١٦) اختناق الرحم يعرض إذا احتبس الطمث وامتلأت الرحم والعروق التي تأتيها ورباطاتها وتمدّدت وتمدّد الرحم إلى فوق ويضغط الحجاب فيضيق النفس وقد يضغط المعدة فيؤلمها ألما شديدا وقد تضغط الأعضاء الموضوعة على الصلب ويؤلمها ألما شديدا. في شرحه لأوجاع النساء.

(17) Sometimes the most likely cause of this illness is the retention of the female sperm and its corruption there [that is, in the uterus]. This was explained at length in the final [book] of *De locis affectis*.[35]

(18) I once saw a woman who had been a widow for a long time. Because[36] of the afflictions she suffered from as a result of hysterical suffocation—for her midwife told me that her uterus had been pulled up—I considered it a good thing that she should use those things for a suppository that are regularly used [for this illness]. But because of the heat of the things used for a suppository and because of the contact of her hand with her genitals during the insertion of the medications, she experienced a spasm together with pain and pleasure, similar to that experienced during sexual intercourse. Immediately after this, thick semen was discharged from her and the woman found relief from all those harmful afflictions. *De locis affectis* 6.[37]

(19) Menstrual blood that flows from a pregnant woman cannot come from the vessels inside the uterus because the placenta is attached to all their openings. Rather, it originates from the vessels in the neck of the uterus. *In Hippocratis Aphorismos commentarius* 6.[38] Similarly, [Galen] mentioned in the last [book] of *De locis affectis* that the blood that flows from pregnant women comes from the bursting of a vessel in the neck of the uterus.[39]

(20) Rapidity of growth in women indicates that their bodies contain a surplus of heat that matches the moisture of their bodies. This is confirmed by the monthly flow of the menstrual blood from their bodies, for when the blood increases the heat increases too. *In Hippocratis De mulierum affectibus commentarius*.[40]

(21) In many pregnant women the uterus often protrudes and prolapses if the labor pains are extremely severe and the expulsive faculty itself is extremely active. This is especially the case when the ligaments connecting the uterus with the spine are naturally weak. *De naturalibus facultatibus* 3.[41]

(١٧) وقد رجح في هذه العلّة أن يكون سببها احتباس منّي المرأة وفساده هناك وطوّل في بيان ذلك في آخر التعرّف.

(١٨) رأيت امرأة أقامت أرملة دهرا طويلا فبسبب ما عرض لها من أعراض اختناق الرحم وبسبب قول القابلة لي أنّ رحمها قد تشمّر إلى فوق رأيت أن تحتمل الأشياء التي قد جرت العادة باستعمالها. فبسبب حرارة تلك الأشياء المحتملة وبسبب ملامسة اليد للفرج عند إدخال الأدوية عرض لها من التشنّج مع وجع ولذّة معا شبيه بما يكون وقت الجماع. وبعقب ذلك خرج منها منّي غليظ واستراحت المرأة من تلك الأعراض المؤذية كلّها. سادسة التعرّف.

(١٩) الطمث الذي يجري من الحامل ليس يمكن أن يخرج من العروق التي داخل الرحم لأنّ المشيمة متعلّقة بأفواه جميعها. وإنّما يكون خروجه من العروق التي في رقبة الرحم. في شرحه لخامسة الفصول وكذلك ذكر في آخر التعرّف أنّ الدم الذي يجري للحوامل هو من انبثاق عروق في عنق الرحم.

(٢٠) سرعة نشء النساء تدلّ على أنّ فيهنّ حرارة زائدة لحقتها رطوبة أبدانهنّ. ويحقّق ذلك ما يجري من أبدانهنّ كلّ شهر من الطمث لأنّ حيث كثر الدم يكثر الحرارة. في شرحه لأوجاع النساء.

(٢١) كثيرا ما يبرز الرحم في كثير من النساء الحوامل فيقع خارجا إذا كان الطلق شديدا جدّا واستعملت القوة الدافعة نفسها بإفراط وخاصّة إذا كانت رباطاته مع عظم الصلب ضعيفة بالطبع. في الثالثة من القوى.

---

١ وقد] قال موسى وقد L || ٣ من أعراض اختناق الرحم وبسبب قول القابلة لي] من الأعراض الآخر بسبب أنّ القابلة قالت W, fol. 164a || ٤ لي] om. L | أعراض] om. B G¹ | لي] om. B G | ٧ منّي] شيء BELOU | كلّها] لها G || ٩ الحامل] الحوامل BELOU | ١١ من] om. G || ١٨ بالطبع] الطبع G

(22) The tumor known as cancer mostly occurs in the breasts of women if their bodies are not cleansed by menstruation. If this cleansing [process] takes place properly, a woman always preserves her health and is not affected by any illness at all. *Ad Glauconem [de methodo medendi]* 2.[42]

(23) A craving for bad foods happens to someone who has bad super-fluities inside the folds of his stomach. This happens to women who have bad humors during their pregnancy. Often they crave anything sour and astringent, or anything acrid or sharp, or clay and charcoal. This happens to most of them until the third month [of their pregnancy]; then it subsides in the fourth month because those [bad] humors are partly evacuated through vomiting and partly concocted during this whole period. For the woman hardly eats anything, since she has no appetite, and by then the fetus feeds itself with substantial things. As a result, the body of the woman is less filled [with foodstuff] and all the bad humors in it are decreased. *De [morborum] causis et symptomatibus* 4.[43]

(24) The symptom[44] of craving bad things, which happens to women, indeed originates from an illness of the cardia of the stomach. All these symptoms that happen to women—a ravenous appetite, or no appetite at all, or only a craving for bad things—all these are [symptoms indicating] diseases affecting the stomach. *De locis affectis* 5.[45]

(25) Male [fetuses] are mostly conceived [by the woman] on the right side of the uterus and female [ones] on the left side. The reverse of this situation only happens rarely. *De locis affectis* 6.[46]

(26) When the breasts of a pregnant woman shrink so much that they become emaciated and thin, you should expect that she will miscarry. If she is pregnant with twins and one of her breasts becomes emaciated and thin, one of her fetuses will be aborted. *De locis affectis* 6.[47]

(27) When a woman conceives and always has a miscarriage after two or three or four months, you should know that this is caused by a phlegmatic moisture that accumulates in the openings[48] of the vessels in the uterus. Depending on the [quantity of] that moisture, the connection of the pulsatile and nonpulsatile vessels in the uterus with the placenta will be weak so that it cannot carry the burden of the fetus but easily tears free from it. *De locis affectis* 6.[49]

(٢٢) الورم المعروف بالسرطان أكثر ما يحدث في الثديين من النساء إذا لم تنقّ أبدانهم بالطمث. و إذا كانت تلك التنقية على ما ينبغي فإنّ المرأة تبقى على صحّتها دائما من غير أن ينالها شيء من الأمراض أصلا. ثانية أغلوقن.

(٢٣) الشهوة للأطعمة الرديئة تعرض لمن يكون في طبقات معدته فضول رديئة مداخلة لها. وهذا يعرض للنساء الرديئات الأخلاط عندما يحبلن. وكثيرا ما يشتهين كلّ شيء حامض ٥ وعفص وكلّ شيء حرّيف حادّ والطين والفحم. ويعرض لأكثرهنّ إلى الشهر الثالث ثمّ يسكن في الرابع لأنّ جزءا من ذلك الخلط يستفرغ بالقيء وجزءا ينضج في طول المدّة لقلّة طعام المرأة لما يعرض لها من ذهاب الشهوة ولأنّ الجنين يغتذي حينئذ بما له قدر. فينقص حينئذ امتلاء بدن المرأة وينقص كلّ ما فيه من الخلط الرديء. رابعة العلل والأعراض.

(٢٤) العلّة التي تعرض للنساء من شهوة الأشياء الرديئة إنّما تعرض بسبب فم المعدة إذا ١٠ اعتلّ. وجميع العلل التي تحدث للنساء عندما يشتهين الشهوة الكلبية أو لا يشتهين أو يشتهين أشياء رديئة كلّ ذلك علل في المعدة. خامسة التعرّف.

(٢٥) الذكور على الأمر الأكثر يحبل بهم في الجانب الأيمن من الرحم والإناث في الجانب الأيسر. ولا يقع الأمر على خلاف ذلك إلّا في الندرة. سادسة التعرّف.

(٢٦) الحامل إذا تكمّشت ثدياها حتّى يهزلان ويقضفان فتوقّع لها أن تسقط. فإن كانت ١٥ حامل بتوأم وتكمّش وقضف أحد الثديين فيسقط واحد من جنينيها. سادسة التعرّف.

(٢٧) إذا كانت المرأة تحبل دائما وتسقط بعد شهرين أو ثلاثة أو أربعة فاعلم أنّ سبب ذلك رطوبة بلغمية تجتمع في أفواه العروق التي في الرحم. وبحسب تلك الرطوبة يكون اتّصال العروق الضوارب وغير الضوارب التي في الرحم بالمشيمة اتّصالا ضعيفا فلا يحتمل ٢٠ ثقل الجنين المحمول بل ينقطع ويتخلّص منه بسهولة. سادسة التعرّف.

---

١ في الثديين] بالثديين ELO ‖ ١٦–١٥ الحامل . . . سادسة التعرّف] om. BE L[1] ‖ ١٦ وقضف] om. OU

(28) During pregnancy the pulse is greater and more frequent and faster. But the other conditions [of the body] remain the same. *De pulsu parva.*[50]

(29) A sign of the wisdom of Nature is that the os uteri is completely closed as long as the fetus within it is alive, but if [the fetus] dies, the os opens to the extent necessary for [it] to make its exit. The midwives do not make the women get up and sit down on the [obstetric] chair during labor pains. But after they have palpated the os uteri when it is gradually dilating—and if it has dilated enough for the fetus to make its exit—they make them sit down on the [obstetric] chair and tell them to expel the fetus by squeezing the muscles in the belly. *De naturalibus facultatibus* 3.[51]

(30) A woman may have a miscarriage because of [excessive] movement or because of taking a bath, for bathing softens the body and the nerves. She may also abort because of excessive anointing of her head because this produces a catarrh. As a result she coughs, the uterus is shaken, and the fetus is expelled. *In Hippocratis De mulierum affectibus commentarius.*[52]

(31) During pregnancy the formative[53] and growth-promoting faculty attracts the best blood to the fetus and leaves the worst blood in the vessels. This blood exits after birth, just like the blood that is quantitatively and qualitatively useless exits every month. *De atra bile.*[54]

(32) The time within which the formation of the fetus is completed is thirty-five or forty or forty-five days. The time within which the fetus begins to move is twice that many days. In three times [the amount] of time within which it moves, the [child] is born. *In Hippocratis De alimento commentarius* 4.[55]

(٢٨) في وقت الحمل يكون النبض أعظم وأشدّ تواترا وأشدّ سرعة. وأمّا سائر الأشياء فتبقى فيه على حالها. في النبض الصغير.

(٢٩) وممّا يدلّ على حكمة الطبيعة أنّ فم الرحم ما دام الطفل فيه حيّا منضمّا انضماما محكما. فإذا مات بلغ من انفتاحه المقدار الذي يحتاج إليه في خروج الجنين. وليس يقمن القوابل أيضا النساء ساعة يصيبهنّ الطلق وتقعدهنّ على كرسي لكنّ بعد أن تلمسن فم الرحم عند انفتاحه قليلا قليلا. فإذا بلغ من انفتاحه المقدار الذي ينبغي به في خروج الجنين أقعدتهنّ على الكرسي وأمرتهنّ بدفع الجنين بعصر عضل البطن. في ثالثة القوى الطبيعية.

(٣٠) قد تسقط المرأة من قِبَل الحركة أو من قِبَل دخول الحمّام لأنّ الحمّام يرخي البدن والعصب. وقد تسقط من قِبَل استعمال الدهن في رأسها بكثرة نزلة فيحدث فتهتزّ الرحم فتطرح الجنين. في شرحه لأوجاع النساء.

(٣١) في حالة الحبل تجذب القوة المصوّرة والمنمّية للجنين أجود الدم وتبقي أرداه في العروق فيخرج بعد الولادة على نحو ما يخرج كلّ شهر ما لا يحتاج إليه من جهة كمّيته أو كيفيته. في مقالته في المرّة السوداء.

(٣٢) الزمان الذي يتمّ فيه خلق الجنين قد يكون خمسة وثلاثين يوما أو أربعين أو خمسة وأربعين وفي ضعف أيّام تكوّنه يتحرّك. والزمان الذي فيه يتحرّك في ثلاثة أضعافه يولد. في شرحه لرابعة الغذاء.

---

٣ حكمة] حركة G | حيّا] فهو ELO || ٤-٧ في . . . ELO | ٧ عضل البطن] من جهة كمّيته أو كيفيته B || في ثالثة القوى الطبيعية] في مقالته في المرّة السودا B || ٨-١٠ قد . . . النساء] om. B | قبل] om.B | قبل] om. ELOU G¹ || ١١-١٢ في . . . الغذاء] om.B | حالة] حال ELOU | الحبل] الحمل EL | الغذاء] ١٦ تمّت المقالة السادسة عشر بحمد الله وعونه وتوفيقه ومنّته add. G

(33) If a woman has a difficult childbirth, the blood that streams during the parturition is mostly retained because the organs of the childbirth swell as a result of the pressure put on them during the difficult delivery. *In Hippocratis Epidemiarum librum* 2 *commentaria* 2.[56]

(34) When a woman gives birth, she needs to evacuate all that corrupt blood that has accumulated during the days of the pregnancy. Her main treatment is the evacuation of that blood. She[57] should be given fluid-promoting food to facilitate the outflow of blood. [A food] both nourishing and moistening is barley [*Hordeum vulgare*] gruel, which, in addition, dilutes and attenuates. It is [a food] that helps the thick blood to flow copiously. *In Hippocratis Epidemiarum librum* 2 *commentaria* 6.[58]

(35) If the milk of the wet nurse is [too thick] or [too thin], it is a warning that an illness will occur.[59] Plenty of [good] milk [in the breasts] indicates that the nature of the breasts is balanced and [they are] capable of [carrying out their] activities. *In Hippocratis De mulierum affectibus commentarius.*[60]

(36) If the milk of a pregnant woman flows copiously, the fetus is weak. Because of its weakness, it does not attract the blood, which recedes to the breasts, and milk is produced. If the breasts are firmer,[61] the fetus is healthier. *In Hippocratis Epidemiarum librum* 2 *commentaria* 6.[62]

(37) The milk of the mother fits the newborn [infant] because its substance is [nothing else but] the substance of the blood from which he was created. If her milk is spoiled, one should choose [other] suitable milk. *In Hippocratis De alimento commentarius* 4.[63]

(38) The accumulation of blood in the breasts indicates that insanity will occur. *In Hippocratis Epidemiarum librum* 2 *commentaria* 6.[64]

This is the end of the sixteenth treatise by the help, guidance, and grace of God, praise be to Him.

(٣٣) إذا عسر على المرأة ولادها فإنّ الدم الذي يجري في وقت النفاس في أكثر الأمر يحتبس عنها لأنّ أعضاء التوليد ترم بسبب الشدّة التي تنالها عند عسر الولادة. في الثانية من شرحه لثانية أبيديميا.

(٣٤) المرأة إذا ولدت تحتاج أن تستفرغ ذلك الدم الفاسد كلّه الذي اجتمع في أيّام الحمل. وملاك هذا الأمر في علاجها استفراغ ذلك الدم وأن تغذى وأن ترطّب كي يسهل درور الدم ومّما يجتمع فيه الغذاء والترطيب ماء كشك الشعير وفيه مع هذا تلطيف وتقطيع. وذلك مّما يعين على درور الدم الثخين. في السادسة من شرحه لثانية أبيديميا.

(٣٥) المرضعة إذا احتبس لبنها أو لم يحتبس بوجه أنذر بمرض. وإن كان غزيرا دلّ على أنّ طبيعة الثديين معتدلة قوية على أفعالها. في شرحه لأوجاع النساء.

(٣٦) الحامل إذا درّ لبنها فالجنين ضعيف ولضعفه لا يجذب الدم ويتراجع إلى الثديين فيتولّد لبن. وإن كان في الثديين فضل اكتناز فالجنين أصحّ. في سادسة شرحه لثانية أبيديميا.

(٣٧) لبن الأمّ موافق للمولود لأنّ جوهره جوهر الدم الذي خلق منه. فإذا فسد لبنها فيختار له لبن موافق. في الرابعة من شرحه للغذاء.

(٣٨) اجتماع الدم في الثديين يدلّ على جنون سيحدث. في سادسة شرحه لثانية أبيديميا.

تمّت المقالة السادسة عشر بحمد اللّه وعونه وتوفيقه ومنّته.

---

١ المرأة] الوالدة L || ٢ ترم] تروم L || ٣ أبيديميا] أفيديميا ELO || ٤ تحتاج] إلى add. EL | كلّه] om. ELO || ٥ هذا] om. ELOU || ٦ ماء] om. G || ٧ أبيديميا] أفيديميا ELO || ٨ يحتبس] يستحكم ELOU || ١٠ الدم] om. ELOU || ١١ أبيديميا] أفيديميا ELO || ١٤ أبيديميا] أفيديميا ELO || ١٥ تمّت المقالة السادسة عشر بحمد اللّه وعونه وتوفيقه ومنّته] تمّت المقالة السادسة عشر والحمد للّه كثيرا كما هو أعلم E تمّت المقالة وعدد فصولها سبعة وثلاثون فصلا B تمّت المقالة L كملت المقالة السادسة عشر الحمد للّه وعدد فصوله سبعة وثلاثون O تمّت المقالة الثامنة لجبيش والحمد للّه وعدد فصولها ستّة وثلثين U

In the name of God,
the Merciful, the Compassionate.
O Lord, make [our task] easy.

The Seventeenth Treatise

Containing aphorisms concerning
the regimen of health in general

(1) Rest is very bad for the maintenance of one's health just as moderate movement is very beneficial. That[1] is, people do not fall ill if they take care that they do not suffer from any bad digestion whatsoever and that they do not strenuously move after eating. Just as exercise before a meal is more beneficial for lasting health than anything else, movement after a meal is more harmful than anything else. *De bonis [malisque] sucis.*[2]

(2) Hippocrates remarks in [book] six of his *Epidemics* that lasting health lies in the avoidance of satiation and in giving up laziness for exertion.[3] Galen says in his first commentary to this statement that the avoidance of overfilling with food is beneficial for all ages and for any bodily condition. *In Hippocratis Epidemiarum librum* 6 *commentaria* 1.[4]

بسم الله الرحمن الرحيم

رب يسّر

المقالة السابعة عشر

تشتمل على فصول تتعلّق

بتدبير الصحّة على العموم

(١) السكون شرّ عظيم في حفظ الصحّة كما أنّ الحركة المعتدلة خير عظيم. وذلك أنّ الإنسان لا يمرض إن هو عني بأن لا يعرض له سوء هضم البتّة ولا يتحرّك بعد الأكل حركة قوية. وكما أنّ الرياضة قبل الطعام أنفع من جميع الأشياء في دوام الصحّة كذلك الحركة بعد الطعام أضرّ من جميع الأشياء. في مقالته في جودة الكيموس.

(٢) قال أبقراط في سادسة أبيديميا: استدامة الصحّة بالتحفّظ من الشبع وترك التكاسل عن التعب. وقال جالينوس في الأولى من شرحه لهذه المقالة: تجنّب الامتلاء من الطعام نافع في كلّ سنّ وفي كلّ حال من أحوال البدن.

١ بسم الله الرحمن الرحيم رب يسّر [om. BELU] || ٣ المقالة السابعة عشر] الصحّة المقالة الثامنة قال حبيش U || ١٠ أبيديميا] أفيديميا ELO || ١٢ سنّ] فنّ EL شيء U

(3) Health is something that all people need. But not everyone is able to follow the regimen that would be appropriate for him, because[5] of gluttony and lust for food, or because he is too busy, or because he does not know what is proper for him to do. *De bonis [malisque] sucis.*[6]

(4) One should not neglect the movement of one's body as scholars do, who diligently study the entire night and day. The body and all its limbs should be moved evenly, and every limb should carry out its activity so that both the internal and external parts of the body receive benefit [therefrom]. *De somno et vigilia.*[7]

(5) To maintain one's health, one should strive after two goals: one, the replacement of that which has dissolved so[8] that it provides the body with something similar and suitable according to its temperament, and the other, the cleansing of the superfluities that unavoidably develop in the body. And a third goal, that one should not age prematurely, is subordinate to the other two goals. *De sanitate tuenda* 1.[9]

(6) One should first of all pay attention to the maintenance of the innate heat, which can be preserved with [different] kinds of moderate exercise for both the body and the soul. *De sanitate tuenda* 1.[10]

(7) For a healthy regimen one should begin by [paying attention to] exercise, then food, then drink, then sleep, and then sexual intercourse. Perform each of these five [activities] to a moderate degree. *In Hippocratis Epidemiarum librum* 6 *commentaria* 6.[11]

(٣) الصحّة أمر يحتاج إليه الناس كلّهم. ولكنْ ليس كلّهم يقدر أن يسوس نفسه السياسة التي ينبغي له إمّا لحال النهم والرغبة وإمّا لكثرة الشغل وإمّا لجهل ما يصلح أن يعمل. في مقالته في جودة الكيموس.

(٤) ينبغي أن لا تغفل عن حركة البدن كما يفعل أهل العلم الذي يكبّون عليه الليل كلّه والنهار. لكنّ ينبغي أن يحرّك البدن والأعضاء كلّها تحريكا مستويا وأن يعمل كلّ عضو عمله فتنتفع أعضاء البدن الداخلة والخارجة. في مقالته في النوم واليقظة.

(٥) الذي ينبغي أن يقصد له في تدبير الصحّة غرضان: أحدهما استخلاف مكان ما يتحلّل حتّى يردّ على البدن ما يشاكله و يوافقه بحسب مزاجه، والغرض الآخر تنقية الفضول التي لا بدّ من تولّدها من البدن. وأمّا الغرض الثالث وهو أن لا يسرع إليه الهرم وهو تابع لذينك الغرضين. الأولى من تدبير الصحّة.

(٦) ينبغي أن تقدم العناية قبل كلّ شيء بحفظ الحرارة الغريزية والذي يتهيّأ به حفظها أصناف الرياضة المعتدلة التي تكون للبدن والنفس جميعا. أولى تدبير الصحّة.

(٧) الذي ينبغي أن تبدأ به في تدبير الصحّة هو الرياضة ثمّ الأطعمة والأشربة ثمّ النوم ثمّ الباه. وتفعل في كلّ واحد من هذه الخمسة المقدار المعتدل. في السادسة من شرحه لسادسة أبيديميا.

٤ الذي] الذين ELOU || ٧ أحدهما] om. BELOU || ٩ من] في EL || ١١ يتهيّأ] يأتي L || ١٢ أولى تدبير الصحّة] في مقالته تلك ELO || ١٥ أبيديميا] أفيديميا ELO

(8) Having sexual intercourse is something that falls under [the category of] the regimen of one's health, meaning that there are intervals between the times in which one has intercourse that one does not feel feeble or weak. Rather [than feeling feeble or weak], one should feel that the body is lighter than before having intercourse.[12] At the time that one has intercourse, one's [body] should not be very full nor very empty nor very cold nor very hot. The same holds true for dryness and moisture. If someone who has intercourse errs in one of these, his error should be [as] small [as possible]; that is, having intercourse with a full or a warm or a moist body is less harmful than doing so in conditions that are opposite to the mentioned ones. *De arte parva*.[13]

(9) Just as sexual intercourse always has a drying effect, it always has a cooling effect. It is beneficial only for him whose body contains a vaporous superfluity because a hot dyscrasia prevails in him by nature. Only in his case is sexual intercourse beneficial, because of its drying and cooling effect. *In Hippocratis Epidemiarum librum* 6 *commentaria* 5.[14]

(10) For the preservation of health one should first of all perform physical exercise; this should be followed by [attending to] food and drink, and then sleep.[15] *De sanitate tuenda* 2.[16]

(11) One should eat after bathing or physical exercise, once the disturbance of the body caused by these [activities] has subsided. Be careful not to take food prior to these [activities] so that it is not transported to the organs before it is digested. If one takes food in a state of disturbance [of the body], it fills the head and usually overflows[17] the cardia of the stomach. *In Hippocratis De acutorum morborum [victu] commentarius* 3.[18]

(12) After a person has exercised properly and has bathed in the prescribed manner and eaten beneficial food and then slept, he can have sexual intercourse if it is appropriate for him. *De sanitate tuenda* 2.[19]

(٨) الجماع من استعماله شيء يدخل في تدبير الصحّة وهو أن يكون بين أوقاته من البعد ما لا يحسّ معه باسترخاء ولا ضعف بل يحسّ أنّ بدنه أخفّ ممّا كان قبل استعماله. ووقت استعماله لا يكون الإنسان ممتلئا جدّا ولا خاويا جدّا ولا قد برد جدّا ولا قد سخن جدّا. وكذلك الحال في اليبس والرطوبة. فإن وقع الخطأ من المستعمل فينبغي أن يكون ذلك الخطأ يسيرا. وذلك أنّ استعماله على الامتلاء أو على حال سخونة البدن أو على حال رطوبته أقلّ ضررا من استعماله على أضداد هذه الحالات. في الصناعة الصغيرة.

(٩) الجماع كما يجفّف دائما كذلك يبرد دائما وإنّما يستنفع به من في بدنه فضل دخاني لغلبة سوء المزاج الحارّ عليه بالطبع. هذا فقط ينفعه الجماع بتجفيفه وتبريده. في الخامسة من شرحه لسادسة أبيديميا.

(١٠) يجب في حفظ الصحّة أن يرتاض الإنسان أوّلا ثمّ يتبع ذلك الطعام والشراب ثمّ يتبع ذلك النوم. ثانية تدبير الصحّة.

(١١) ينبغي أن يتناول الغذاء بعد الاستحمام أو الرياضة بعد سكون الاضطراب الحادث في البدن عنها. واحذر أن تتناول الغذاء قبلها لأن لا ينصرف إلى الأعضاء قبل انهضامه. وتناوله في حال الاضطراب يملأ الرأس ويطفو في فم المعدة في أكثر الأمر. في شرحه لثالثة الأمراض الحادّة.

(١٢) بعد أن يرتاض الإنسان على ما ينبغي ويستحمّ على ما ذكر ويغتذي بما يصلح وينام بعد ذلك يجامع إن كان الجماع موافقا له. ثانية تدبير الصحّة.

---

١ من] في ELO || ٥ حال] om. ELO || ٨ هذا فقط] om. EL || ٩ أبيديميا] أفيديميا ELO || ١٠ يجب] ينبغي ELO || ١٢ يتناول] يكون G || ١٦ على ما] كما BELOU

(13) Only someone with a hot and moist body or someone with a body in which much sperm is naturally produced is free from the harm caused by sexual intercourse. But the harm it causes to someone whose temperament tends towards dryness or to old people is very severe. *De sanitate tuenda* 6.[20]

(14) Some bodily constitutions are very bad. That is, in some people much hot, biting sperm is produced, which stimulates them to eject it. If they do so during sexual intercourse, the cardia of their stomach becomes flaccid as does their whole body; they become weak and dry and lean; their complexion changes and their eyes sink in. But if they abstain from sexual intercourse, their head becomes heavy and they suffer from pain in their stomach. Abstaining from sexual intercourse harms them just as much as having sexual intercourse.[21]

As to the regimen of these people, my advice is that they abstain from anything producing sperm, consume foods and medications that suppress its formation, and exercise the upper parts of their body by playing with a small or large ball or by lifting stones. After bathing he[22] should anoint his loins with cooling oils. If he wants to expel the sperm, he should feed himself with good foodstuff during that day, and in the evening, when he wants to go to sleep, he should have sexual intercourse and then go to sleep. When he wakes up on the following day, his body should be massaged with linen cloths until the skin becomes red, and then he should be moderately rubbed with oil. He should wait a little while and then eat solid[23] bread steeped in diluted wine. Then he should go about his affairs. *De sanitate tuenda* 6.[24]

(15) I advise all people to abstain from all foods that produce bad humors. Even if someone digests them easily and rapidly, he should not be misled by this because undoubtedly a bad humor will accumulate in his vessels even though he does not notice. It will putrefy from the slightest cause, and from this malignant fevers will arise. *De alimentorum [facultatibus]* 2.[25]

(16) One[26] acts prudently and securely when [one takes care] that the passages and channels of the food through the liver are open and clean, not only in the case of sick people but also [in the case of] healthy people. *De alimentorum [facultatibus]* 2.[27]

(١٣) لا يسلم من ضرر الجماع إلّا من كان بدنه حارًّا رطبا أو كان بالطبع يتولّد فيه المنيّ كثيرا ومضرّته بمن مزاجه مائل إلى اليبس أو الشيوخ عظيمة. سادسة تدبير الصحّة.

(١٤) قد توجد هيئات رديئة جدًّا من هيئات البدن وهي أنّ قوما يتولّد فيهم منيّ كثير حارّ لذّاع يهيجهم لنفضه فإذا نفضوه بالجماع استرخى فم المعدة منهم واسترخى بدنهم بجملته وضعفوا وجفّوا ونحفوا وتغيّرت ألوانهم وغارت أعينهم. فإن امتنعوا من الجماع ثقلت روسهم وتكرّبوا من معدهم ويعرض لهم من منع الجماع ضرر مثل ما يعرض لهم من الجماع.

وتدبير هؤلاء عندي أن يمتنعوا من كلّ ما يولّد المنيّ ويتناولوا أطعمة وأدوية تطفئ المنيّ ويروضوا أعالي أبدانهم بلعب الكرة الصغيرة أو الكبيرة أو شيل الأحجار. ويمسح القطن بعد الاستحمام بأدهان مبرّدة. وإذا همّ بنفض المنيّ يغتذي ذلك اليوم بغذاء محمود فإذا تعشّى وهمّ بالنوم يجامع وينام وإذا انتبه من الغد دلك بدنه بمناديل حتّى يحمرّ الجلد، ثمّ يمرخ بالدهن مرخا معتدلا، ثمّ يمسك قليلا ويأكل خبزا محكم الصنعة منقوعا في خمرة ممزوجة، ثمّ يتصرّف في أشغاله. سادسة تدبير الصحّة.

(١٥) أشير على جميع الناس أن يجتنبوا جميع الأغذية المولّدة للأخلاط الرديئة ولو أنّ الرجل استمرأها بسهولة وسرعة فلا يغتّر بذلك فلا بدّ أن تجتمع في عروقه وهو لا يشعر خلط رديء يعفن بأيسر سبب وتحدث عنه حمّيات خبيثة. ثانية الأغذية.

(١٦) من الحزم والعمل بالوثيقة أن تكون منافذ الغذاء ومجاريه من الكبد مفتوحة نقية لا في المرضى فقط لكنّ في الأصحّاء أيضا. ثانية الأغذية.

١–٢ لا يسلم ... سادسة تدبير الصحّة [om. B ‖ ٢ أو الشيوخ [وبالشيوخ ELOU ‖ ٣ قد [om. BELOU ‖ ٥ وضعفوا [om. ELOU ‖ ٩ يغتذي [بعد add. G ‖ ١٢ سادسة [سابعة ELU ‖ ١٦ من [om. ELO ‖ من [في L ‖ ١٧ ثانية الأغذية [في مقالته تلك EL

(17) A good regimen is beneficial for the soul and bestows it with excellent ethical qualities, just as it is salutary for the body and provides it with health. This is especially true if a person adheres to a good regimen immediately after being born. *De sanitate tuenda* 1.[28]

(18) One's moral character is impaired by bad habits in food, drink, exercise, sights, and sounds.[29] Bad[30] humors often cause diseases. *De sanitate tuenda* 1.[31]

(19) The first thing to consider regarding anyone's regimen of health is the calculation of the times of nourishment, whether you should let him eat once or twice [a day], depending on his temperament.[32] Some bilious persons should eat three times [a day]. Be extremely careful that one does not suffer from constipation, but that one's stools tend slightly towards softness.[33] *De sanitate tuenda* 6.

(20) I advise all educated[34] people not to follow the regimen of most people who behave as dumb animals in seeking that which is most pleasurable and nothing else. Rather, every person should test by experience what foods, drinks, and activities[35] are harmful for him and consequently avoid them. Similarly, he should test whether sexual intercourse is harmful and [if so], after how much time it is no longer harmful. His regimen in this matter should be thus: he should look and strive for all that is beneficial for him and avoid all that is harmful to him. Anyone who follows such a regimen has little need for a physician, as long as he is healthy. *De sanitate tuenda* 6.[36]

(21) If someone needs additional nourishment, he should be given moist food in the morning, such as broth, and dry food in the evening, such as bread and meat. There are three [kinds of] dry foods: seeds, parts of plants, and parts of animals. *In Hippocratis De alimento commentarius* 1.[37]

(١٧) من شأن التدبير المحمود أن ينفع النفس ويكسبها أخلاقا محمودة كما ينفع البدن ويكسبه صحّة ولا سيّما إن تدبّر الإنسان بالتدبير المحمود من أوّل ما يولد. الأولى من تدبير الصحّة.

(١٨) الفساد يعرض في الأخلاق من اعتياد الأشياء الرديئة في المطعم والمشرب وفي الرياضة وفي مشاهدة ما يشاهد وفي سماع ما يسمع. وكثيرا ما تكون الأخلاط الرديئة أسبابا للأمراض. الأولى من تدبير الصحّة.

(١٩) الذي تقدمه في النظر في تدبير الصحّة في كلّ شخص تقدير أوقات الغذاء إن تجعل طعامه مرّة واحدة أو مرّتين بحسب مزاجه. ومن أرباب المرار من يأكل طعامه في ثلاث مرّات. والعناية كلّ العناية بالطبع أن لا يحتبس ويميل إلى اللين قليلا. سادسة تدبير الصحّة.

(٢٠) أنا أشير على كافّة الفضلاء أن لا يتدبّروا بتدبير الكثير من الناس الذي يتدبّروا تدبير البهائم وهو طلب الألذّ لا غير. بل ينبغي لكلّ شخص أن يمتحن بالتجربة أيّ الأطعمة وأيّ الأشربة وأيّ الحركات تضرّه فيجتنبها. وكذلك يجرّب الجماع هل يضرّه وبعد كم من الزمان لا يضرّه. ويتدبّر فيه بحسب ذلك ويفتقد كلّ ما ينفعه فيقصده وكلّ ما يضرّه فيجتنبه. فإنّ من تدبّر هكذا قلّت حاجته للأطبّاء ما دام صحيحا. سادسة تدبير الصحّة.

(٢١) من يحتاج الزيادة في الغذاء فينبغي أن يعطى بالغداة غذاء رطبا مثل الحسو وبالعشي غذاء يابسا مثل الخبز واللحم. والأغذية اليابسة ثلاثة: البزور وأجزاء النبات وأجزاء الحيوان. في شرحه للأولى من الغذاء.

---

٧ الصحّة في [om. BELOU | إن [هل [ELOU لـ B- || ٨ أرباب [أصحاب L || ٩ كلّ العناية [om. L ||
١٠ أنا [om. ELO | يتدبّروا [يتدبّر ELOU

(22) Well-prepared[38] barley groats are better than all the other foods for [producing] good chyme and for the preservation of health. It is no less nourishing than the nourishment of good bread. *De bonis [malisque] sucis.*[39]

(23) In seeking health, a bad but regular diet of food and drink is more reliable, safer, and farther removed from danger than if a person suddenly replaces his diet with something else that is better.[40] There are things that are by nature peculiar to some people and similar to their nature while other things are not peculiar to them and not similar to their nature.[41] *De usis.*[42]

(24) I have seen many people who, although the regimen they followed was not at all good in all the other aspects, yet ended up healthy by [the ingestion of] squill [*Urginea maritima*] vinegar and squill wine. *De victu attenuante.*[43]

(25) Rockfish is rapidly digested. Together with its high digestibility, it is extremely good and beneficial in preserving the health of a human body since it produces blood of an intermediate consistency, neither thin and fine nor thick. *De alimentorum [facultatibus]* 3.[44]

(26) Children should not be allowed to taste wine for a long time, for wine is very harmful to them. It moistens and heats their bodies more than necessary, fills their heads [with vapors], and corrupts the ethical qualities of their souls. *De sanitate tuenda* 1.[45]

It is not good for [adult] persons to drink more than a moderate amount of wine, because it rapidly brings a person to anger, indecency, and obscene language and makes the rational part of his soul confused and his subtle mind sluggish. *De sanitate tuenda* 1.[46]

(٢٢) كشك الشعير المحكم الصنعة أفضل من سائر الأطعمة في جودة كيموسه وفي حفظ الصحّة وهو يغذو غذاء ليس بدون غذاء الخبز الجيّد. في مقالته في جودة الكيموس.

(٢٣) التدبير الرديء في المطعم والمشرب المعتاد أوثق وأحرز وأبعد عن الخطر في التماس الصحّة من أن ينقل الرجل تدبيره دفعة إلى شيء آخر أفضل. وثمّ بالطبع أشياء خاصّية لقوم مشاكلة لطبائعهم وأشياء غير خاصّية لهم ولا مشاكلة لطبائعهم. في مقالته في العادات. ٥

(٢٤) رأيت خلقا كثيرا وإن كانوا في سائر تدبيرهم لم يتدبّروا تدبيرا جيّدا جدّا صاروا مصحّحين بخلّ العنصل وشراب العنصل. في مقالته في التدبير الملطّف.

(٢٥) السمك الصخري سريع الانهضام ومع سرعة انهضامه هو في غاية الجودة والموافقة لحفظ صحّة بدن الإنسان من قبل أنّه يولّد دما متوسّط القوام ليس باللطيف الدقيق ولا بالغليظ. ثالثة الأغذية. ۱۰

(٢٦) لا يطلق للصبيان أن يذوقوا الخمر إلى مدّة طويلة فإنّه يضرّهم مضرّة عظيمة، يرطّب أبدانهم ويسخنها بأكثر ممّا ينبغي ويملأ رؤوسهم ويفسد أخلاق النفس منهم. الأولى من تدبير الصحّة.

ليس بجيّد للرجال أن يشربوا من الخمر أكثر من المقدار القصد. وذلك أنّها تخرج الرجل إلى سرعة الغضب وإلى الفحش والحنى وتكدّر الفكر من النفس وتكسر حدّة الذكاء. الأولى ۱٥ من تدبير الصحّة.

---

۲ غذاء [om. G ‖ ۳ أوثق [أوفق GL ‖ وأحرز [om. L ‖ ٤ لقوم [= Greek text τισὶν) تقوم B om. (= ed. Klein-Franke) ‖ ٦ سائر [om. BELOU ‖ ۱۱–۱۳ لا ... الأولى من تدبير الصحّة [om. ELOU ‖ أن [om. G

(27) In general, the regimen of health of the elderly should consist of massage with oil in the morning after sleep, followed by walking or slow riding, bathing in hot sweet water, drinking wine, and the consumption of heating and moistening foods. *De sanitate tuenda* 5.[47]

(28) Just as wine is extremely harmful for children, so for the elderly it is extremely beneficial. The wine that is most salutary for them is warm and thin and has a bright reddish color. It is the one that Hippocrates calls "tawny." *De sanitate tuenda* 5.[48]

(29) Let a weak old person eat three times a day, for when his strength is weak, he should be nourished by small amounts at short intervals.[49] And when his strength is great, he should be nourished with large quantities of food at long intervals.[50] *De sanitate tuenda* 5.

(30) Bread for the elderly should be perfectly[51] baked. Milk is not beneficial for all old people but only for those who can digest it well and in whom no flatulence[52] develops in the hypochondria. *De sanitate tuenda* 5.[53]

(31) Let old people eat ripe fresh figs [*Ficus carica*]. Prefer these above other fruits.[54] But in the winter [give them] dried figs.[55] *De sanitate tuenda* 5.[56]

(32) Watery phlegmatic superfluities have the property of accumulating and increasing in the [bodies] of the elderly; therefore, it is necessary to stimulate micturition daily, not with drugs but with celery [*Apium graveolens* and var.], honey, and wines. Their stools should be softened, above all with olive oil, which they should drink before meals.[57] Similarly, one should give them a clyster with olive oil only,[58] and they should take vegetables with olive oil and garum before meals,[59] or plums [*Prunus domestica* var.] boiled with honey.[60] *De sanitate tuenda* 5.

(٢٧) تدبير صحّة الشيوخ على العموم بالدلك بالدهن بالغداة بعد النوم، ثمّ المشي أو الركوب برفق والاستحمام بالماء الحارّ العذب وشرب الخمر وتناول الأطعمة المسخنة المرطّبة. خامسة تدبير الصحّة.

(٢٨) كما أنّ الصبيان تضرّهم الخمر غاية المضرّة كذلك المشائخ ينتفعون بها غاية المنفعة. ويصلح لهم من الخمور ما كان أشدّ حرارة وأميل إلى الرقّة ولونه أحمر ناصع وهو الذي يسمّيه أبقراط كوصيا. خامسة تدبير الصحّة.

(٢٩) اجعل ما يتناوله الشيخ الضعيف من الغذاء في ثلاث مرّات بالنهار لأنّ القوة متى كانت ضعيفة فينبغي أن يغذى قليلا قليلا في ما بين مدد قصيرة. ومتى كانت قوية *غذيته بغذاء كثير في ما بين مدد طويلة. خامسة تدبير الصحّة.

(٣٠) خبز الشيوخ الخبز المحكم الصنعة وليس يصلح اللبن لجميع الشيوخ بل لمن يستمرئه استمراء جيّدا ولا يحدث له نفخ في ما دون الشراسيف. خامسة تدبير الصحّة.

(٣١) تطعم الشيوخ من التين الطريء ما قد نضج منه وتؤثره على سائر الفاكهة وفي الشتاء من التين اليابس. خامسة تدبير الصحّة.

(٣٢) من شأن الفضول البلغمية المائية أن تجتمع وتكثر في بدن الشيوخ فينبغي أن يدرّ بولهم في كلّ يوم لا بالأدوية بل بالكرفس والعسل والخمور وتلان بطونهم بالزيت خاصّة يتحسّى قبل الطعام. وكذلك يحقن به وحده ويتناولون البقول بالزيت والمرّي قبل الطعام أو الإجّاص المطبوخ بالعسل. خامسة تدبير الصحّة.

---

٦ كوصيا .om B خوصيا G خواصيا EL (* = كرصيا = κιρρός) ‖ ٨ *غذيته (= P, fol.27b) غذيت MSS ‖ ١٠ يصلح .om ELO اللبن] جيد add. L ‖ ١١ خامسة تدبير الصحّة] في مقالته تلك ELO ‖ ١٣ خامسة تدبير الصحّة] في مقالته تلك ELO ‖ ١٦ وكذلك . . . قبل الطعام] .om ELO

(33) Of any food or drink, one should first consume [things] that soften the stools, like sweet wines and softening vegetables prepared with olive oil and garum. After the meal one should consume astringent foods to strengthen the cardia of the stomach. *De sanitate tuenda* 6.[61]

(34) For the elderly and those with weak bodies, slaughter the animal a day and a night before cooking it and then cook it well. But for young people and for those who have strong bodies and for workers and heavy laborers, boil fresh meat, but do let it become well done during the roasting or cooking. *In Hippocratis De alimento commentarius* 4.[62]

(35) Old age has three stages: the first stage, that[63] in which old age has just begun, is one in which a person is [still] able to carry out his civic affairs. The[64] second stage is that in which the elderly should follow the regimen mentioned [before]. The third stage, the age of senility,[65] is that in which a person who is in that stage does not tolerate bathing every day, and[66] in which sharp biting [superfluities] do not accumulate in his body. *De sanitate tuenda* 5.[67]

(36) To avert or prevent old age is something impossible. However, it is possible to prevent it from arriving rapidly, and this can be accomplished with a [fitting] diet, frequent bathing, sleeping on a soft bed, and avoiding everything that dries or cools. *De marcore*.[68]

(37) We know that some people suffer from regularly recurring nosebleeds, that others evacuate blood from the vessels in the buttocks, and others when emesis or diarrhea happens to them, and that [yet others] evacuate blood through venesection or by making an incision[69] or by emptying their bodies through purgatives.[70] When their usual manner of evacuation is discontinued, they fall ill because their regimen is a bad one. Therefore, bad humors accumulate in their bodies, which unless they are expelled by the activity of nature—whether spontaneous or provoked—remain in their bodies and make them ill.[71] But when

(۳۳) ينبغي أن يقدم أوّلا بين جميع ما يؤكل و يشرب ما كان مليّنا للطبيعة كالخمور الحلوة والبقول المليّنة المتّخذة بالزيت والمرّي. ويتناول بعد الطعام الأطعمة العفصة لتقوية فم المعدة. سادسة تدبير الصحّة.

(۳٤) الشيوخ وأصحاب الأبدان الضعيفة تذبح لهم الحيوان قبل طبخه بيوم وليلة و ينضج طبخه. والشابّ وأصحاب الأبدان القوية والفعلة وأصحاب الأعمال القوية تطبخ لهم اللحوم الطريئة ولا تنضج لهم جيّدا في الشيّ أو الطبخ. في الرابعة شرحه للغذاء.

(۳٥) الشيخوخة ثلاثة أجزاء والجزء الأوّل وهو القريب العهد بالشيخوخة يمكن الإنسان أن يتصرّف فيه في تصرّفات المدن. وجزؤها الثاني هو الذي يدبّر فيه الشيخ كما ذكر. وجزؤها الثالث وهو سنّ الهرم لا يحتمل من كان فيه الاستحمام كلّ يوم ولا يجتمع في بدنه ما هو حادّ لذّاع. خامسة تدبير الصحّة.

(۳٦) دفع الشيخوخة ومنعها ممّا لا يمكن أن يكون. وأمّا المنع من السرعة فيها فممكن وذلك بما يدبّر به الشيوخ في أغذيتهم وكثرة الاستحمام والنوم والفراش اللّين والتحفّظ من كلّ ما يجفّف أو يبرد. في مقالته في الذبول.

(۳۷) قد نعلم أنّ قوما يصيبهم الرعاف بأدوار في أوقات متساوية وقوما آخرين يستفرغ منهم الدم من العروق التي في السفلة. وقوم آخرون يستفرغون بالقيء أو باختلاف يصيبهم وقوم يستفرغون بالفصد أو بالشرط أو يفرّغون أبدانهم بأدوية مسهلة. ومتى يعطل عنهم ذلك الاستفراغ المعتاد مرضوا لأنّ تدبيرهم تدبيرا رديئا فتجتمع في أبدانهم الأخلاط الرديئة التي إن لم تخرج بفعل الطبيعة دون استدعاء أو باستدعاء بقيت في أبدانهم وأمرضتهم. ومتى

٥ والشابّ] والشباب BELOU || ٦ جيّدا] جدّا EL || ٩ ذكر] ذكرنا BELOU | سنّ] جزء L || ١١ ومنعها ممّا] G¹ || ١٤ نعلم] أعلم BELOU || ١٨ إن] om. BE | بفعل] لفعل B | ومتى ما .add BELOU

those who use these evacuations change their regimen and eat less food and increase their physical exercise, they are safe from illness, for a change in habit at that time is something that is beneficial for them.[72] *De usis.*

(38) I do not advise giving the elderly any aloe [*Aloe vera*] or *hiera.*[73] If they suffer from constipation for two days, it is sufficient to soften their stools with lesser[74] bindweed [*Convolvulus arvensis*], or olive oil, or safflower [*Carthamus tinctorius*] hearts with barley groats, or with the hearts of dried figs and safflower, or with the amount of one or two hazelnuts[75] of resin from the terebinth tree [*Pistacia terebinthus*]. For this remedy softens the stools without harm, purges the intestines, and cleanses what is in the liver, spleen, kidneys, urinary bladder, and lungs. One should use these [laxatives] variously so that nature does not get used to one particular laxative and consequently become resistant to it. *De sanitate tuenda* 5.[76]

(39) If[77] someone complains of constant headache because of hypersensitivity of the nerves that spread in the cardia of the stomach, its treatment is a matter of the art of the regimen of health. That is, he should hasten to take food every day before the bile flows into the stomach, and he should change his diet to a cooler and moister one. If bile streams into the stomach, it should be evacuated through emesis and through purging the belly downwards. For drugs he should use, at long intervals, absinthe wormwood [*Artemisia absinthium* and var.] and the *picra*[78] remedy. His stomach should be anointed externally with quince [*Cydonia oblonga*] oil and nard[79] oil and similar slightly astringent oils. *De sanitate tuenda* 6.[80]

(40) If food putrefies in the stomach and the putrefied material is passed [through the bowels], it is most beneficial for the preservation of health. But if it is not passed, it should be promoted by that which passes it without biting or harm, such as the cumin[81] stomachic, or the remedy

أبدل أصحاب هذه الاستفراغات تدبيرهم وقلّلوا طعامهم وزادوا في رياضتهم سلموا من الأمراض فتتبدّل العادة حينئذ ممّا ينتفع به. في مقالته في العادات.

(٣٨) لست أشير أن يعطى الشيخ شيئا من الصبر أو الإيارج. فإن احتبست الطبيعة منهم يومين فيكتفي في تليينها باللبلاب الصغير أو الزيت أو لباب القرطم مع كشك الشعير أو بلبّ التين اليابس والقرطم أو بمقدار جِلَّوْزَة أو جلوزتين من صمغ البطم فإنّه يلين البطن من غير أذى وينقّي الأحشاء ويجلو ما في الكبد والطحال والكليتين والمثانة والرئة. ويستعمل من هذه هذا مرّة وهذا مرّة حتّى لا تألف الطبيعة الشيء الواحد فلا تتأثّر له. خامسة تدبير الصحّة.

(٣٩) من يشكو دائما الصداع بسبب كثرة حسّ العصب المنبثّ في فم المعدة فعلاجه داخل في صناعة تدبير الصحّة. وذلك بأن يبادر في كلّ يوم بتناول الطعام قبل أن تنصبّ المرار إلى المعدة ويصرف التدبير كلّه إلى التبريد والترطيب. وإن انصبّ مرار إلى المعدة استفرغ بالقيء وإحدار البطن ويستعمل من الأدوية في ما بين مدد طويلة الأفسنتين ودواء الفيقرا وتدهن المعدة من خارج بدهن السفرجل ودهن الناردين ونحوها من الأدهان القابضة قبضا يسيرا. سادسة تدبير الصحّة.

(٤٠) متى فسد الطعام في المعدة وانحدر ما فسد كان ذلك من أفضل الغنائم في بقاء الصحّة. وإن لم ينحدر يعان على انحداره بما يحدر من غير لذع ولا أذى كالجوارشن الكمّوني

٥

١٠

١٥

---

prepared with dried figs and safflower hearts, or other [remedies] prepared with safflower and epithyme [*Cuscuta epithymum*]. The patient also benefits from vomiting the putrefied material. *De sanitate tuenda* 6.[82]

(41) Galen advises that he who takes the theriac[83] to preserve his health should do so once the food has been digested and left the stomach. One should take an amount of it equal to the size of an Egyptian[84] bean in two spoons of water. If one needs an amount equal to a hazelnut, one should dilute it with three spoons of water. Do not take it in the summertime, and no young person nor someone with a hot temperament [should consume it]. But if one resorts to it [in such a case] because of an emergency, it should be a small amount. In the case of children, one should be extremely cautious in administering it to them. He mentioned [the case of] a man who forced a son of his, while still a child, to drink [some] theriac, and when the boy had taken this medicine, his nature could not transform it. As a result [the theriac] dissolved his body and made him suffer from diarrhea, and the boy died that very night. Similarly, he advised that the elderly and old people, if they take it, should dilute it with wine, not with water. *De theriaca ad Pisonem.*[85]

This is the end of the seventeenth treatise, by the grace of God, praise be to Him.

والدواء المتّخذ بتين يابس ولبّ قرطم وسائر ما يتّخذ بالقرطم والأفتيمون. وينتفع أيضا بقيء ما قد فسد. سادسة تدبير الصحّة.

(٤١) جالينوس أشار على من يأخذ الترياق لتدبير الصحّة أن يأخذه بعد انهضام الطعام وخروجه عن المعدة وأن يأخذ منه قدر باقلّي مصرية بملعقتي ماء. وإذا احتيج لمقدار بندقة فيداف ثلاث ملاعق ماء. وأن لا يؤخذ في زمان الصيف ولا يشرب به لا شابّ ولا محرور المزاج. ٥ وإن التجأ إلى ذلك لضرورة فقدر يسير ويحذر منه الغلمان جدّا جدّا. وذكر أنّ رجلا قهر ابنا له غلاما على شرب الترياق فلما شرب الغلام الدواء لم تقو طبيعته على تغيّره فحلّل بدنه وأطلق بطنه ومات الغلام في ليلته تلك. وكذلك أشار على الكهول والشيوخ إذا تناولوه أن يديفوه في الخمر لا في الماء. في مقالته في الترياق إلى قيصر.

تمّت المقالة السابعة عشر بحمد الله ومنّته. ١٠

---

٢ تدبير الصحّة . . . في مقالته تلك [ELO || ١٠ تمّت المقالة السابعة عشر بحمد الله ومنّته] تمّت المقالة السابعة عشر وعدد فصولها واحد وأربعون فصلا والحمد لله كثيرا E تمّت المقالة وعدد فصولها واحد وأربعون فصلا L تمّت المقالة السابعة عشر B تمّت المقالة والحمد لله على حسن عونه O تمّت المقالة التاسعة لجيش الحمد ‹لله› U | ومنّته] تتلو بها المقالة الثامنة عشر .add G

In the name of God,
the Merciful, the Compassionate.
O Lord, make [our task] easy.

The Eighteenth Treatise

Containing aphorisms concerning physical exercise

(1) If someone is able to exercise before meals, he[1] does not have to be very careful [about his diet]. But if someone's occupations distract him from exercise, a healthy diet alone is only sufficient if it is combined with the ingestion of drugs that promote health. *De [bonis malisque] sucis.*[2]

(2) The most beneficial of all types of exercise is that which is able not only to exert the body, but also to gladden and delight the soul, such as hunting and ball playing. For the motion of the soul is so powerful that many have been released from their diseases simply by the pleasure that they experienced. And[3] many, on the other hand, were released from diseases caused by harm inflicted on their soul. *De parvae pilae exercitio.*[4]

بسم اللّه الرحمن الرحيم

ربّ يسّر

المقالة الثامنة عشر

تشتمل على فصول تتعلّق بالرياضة

(١) من يمكنه الرياضة قبل الطعام فليس يحتاج إلى التحفّظ الشديد. وأمّا من تشغله

أشغال عن الرياضة فليس تجزيه جودة التدبير وحده حتّى ينضاف لذلك تناول الأدوية

الصحّية. في مقالته في الكيموس.

(٢) أفضل أنواع الرياضة ما أمكن فيه مع إتعاب البدن أن تسرّ النفس وتفرح كالصيد

واللعب بالكرّة. فإنّ لحركة النفس من القوة ما قد بلغ من مقدارها أنّ قوما كثيرين أقلعت

عنهم الأمراض بفرح فرحوه فقط. وقوم كثير أقلعت عنهم أمراضهم من جهة أخرى بسبب

أذى نال أنفسهم. في مقالته في اللعب بالكرة الصغيرة.

٥

١٠

---

١ بسم اللّه الرحمن الرحيم ربّ يسّر] om. BELU بسم اللّه الرحمن الرحيم O ‖ ٣ المقالة الثامنة عشر]
المقالة الثالثة عشر O الرياضة المقالة التاسعة قال حبيش U ‖ ٦ عن] om. B ‖ ٩ لحركة] بحركة ELO ‖
١٠ كثير] كثيرون L كثيرين BOU | من جهة أخرى] om. L | بسبب أخر EO ‖ ١١ نال أنفسهم] كان
(قد) G¹ نال اكثرهم(؟) G

38 ۞ ٣٨

(3) One should pay more attention to the motions of the soul than to those of the body, as the soul has eminence over the body. In all kinds of exercise one should strive after a combination of exertion with joy, pleasure, and gladness. This can be achieved most easily by playing with a small ball that the players throw from hand to hand.[5] *De parvae pilae exercitio.*[6]

One aspect in which exercise with the small ball is superior to the other types of exercise is that with this [kind of exercise] one can move all the parts of the body [together], or move some part to the exclusion of another. It can also be practiced quietly and gently or vigorously and strenuously as long as no danger or harm ensues afterward, as is the case with most of the other types of exercise. *De parvae pilae exercitio.*[7]

(4) The application of physical exercise is more successful [than other means of evacuation] because it evacuates that[8] which is spread deep in the body, [both] in the flesh and in the parts that are more solid than flesh. *In Hippocratis Aphorismos commentarius* 3.[9]

(5) If someone does not perform physical exercise, both thick and thin humors accumulate in his body: the thick ones because of ease of life and restfulness and the thin and watery ones because he misses their evacuation through exercise. *In Hippocratis Epidemiarum librum* 3 *commentaria* 3.[10]

(6) Physical exercise should not be practiced at all after the poor digestion [of food]. *De sanitate tuenda* 3.[11]

(7) If someone happens to exercise with a body that is full of phlegm or yellow bile or black bile or blood, it results in epilepsy or apoplexy or other [afflictions] because it dissolves the humors and moves them to the outer side [of the body]. *In Hippocratis Aphorismos commentarius* 3.[12]

(٣) ينبغي أن تجرّد العناية بأمر حركات النفس أكثر من العناية بأمر حركات البدن بحسب شرف النفس على البدن. ويقصد في جميع أنواع الرياضة أن يجتمع فيها لصاحبها مع التعب سرور ونزهة وفرح. وأسهل شيء ينال به ذلك اللعب بالكرّة الصغيرة التي يرموها اللاعبون بها من يد إلى يد. في تلك المقالة.

من فضيلة الرياضة بالكرّة الصغيرة على سائر أنواع الرياضة أنّها يمكنك فيها أن تحرّك الأعضاء كلّها. ويمكن أن يحرّك بعضها دون بعض ويمكن أن يرتاض بها رياضة ساكنة ضعيفة أو رياضة قوية شديدة ولا يعقبها شيء من أنواع الخطر والآفات التي تتبع جلّ أنواع الرياضة. في تلك المقالة.

(٤) الرياضة أنجح ما يستعمل لأنّها تستفرغ ما في عمق البدن منبثًّا في اللحم وفي الأعضاء التي هي أصلب من اللحم. في شرحه لثالثة الفصول.

(٥) من لا يستعمل الرياضة تجتمع في بدنه أخلاط غليظة ورقيقة. أمّا الغليظة فللخفض والدعة وأمّا الرقيقة المائية فلفقده الاستفراغ بالرياضة. في ثالثة شرحه لثالثة أبيديميا.

(٦) ليس ينبغي أن تستعمل الرياضة أصلا بعقب سوء الاستمراء. ثالثة تدبير الصحّة.

(٧) الرياضة إذا صادفت البدن مملوءًا من البلغم أو من المرّة الصفراء أو السوداء أو الدم حدث على صاحبه منها إمّا صرع وإمّا سكتة وإمّا غير ذلك لأنّها تذيب الفضول وتحرّكها للخروج. في شرحه لثالثة الفصول.

(8) If someone indulges excessively in idleness, two kinds of overfilling develop in his body as a result: that which pertains to the vessels and that which pertains to the strength [of the body]. *In Hippocratis De natura hominis commentarius.*[13]

(9) Strenuous physical exercise dries the body and makes it hard and slow of sensation and understanding. Therefore, wrestlers and those who carry heavy burdens and stones are ignorant and have little understanding. *De somno et vigilia.*[14]

(10) Extremely hot bodies do not need physical exercise at all. For them walking, bathing, and good[15] rubbing with oil is sufficient. Bathing is beneficial to them after [having] food. *De sanitate tuenda* 6.[16]

(11) Old people need to move their bodies because their heat needs to be fanned. But no elderly person should rest and repose completely so that he does not move at all. On the other hand, he does not need brisk exercise, because brisk exercise cools and extinguishes their heat, which is [already] weak [by itself]. *De sanitate tuenda* 5.[17]

(12) The definition of physical exercise is a vigorous movement that changes respiration. When a person makes any movement that forces him to breathe stronger, faster, and more frequently than before, such a movement becomes exercise for that person. *De sanitate tuenda* 2.[18]

(13) The best time for physical exercise is after the food of the previous day has been completely acted upon and digested in the stomach and vessels and it is time for the next meal. An indication for this is a moderately yellow urine and the expulsion of all [the superfluities] retained in the bladder and the lower intestines. Thereafter, recommend physical exercise. *De sanitate tuenda* 2.[19]

(٨) من أفرط في الخفض تولّد في بدنه من ذلك جنسا الامتلاء جميعا يعني الامتلاء الذي بحسب الأوعية والامتلاء الذي بحسب القوة. في شرحه لطبيعة الإنسان.

(٩) الرياضة القوية تيبّس البدن وتصيره جاسيا، بطيء الحسّ بطيء الفهم ولذلك صاروا المصارعون وأصحاب الأحمال الثقيلة والذين يشيلون الحجارة جهّالا قليلة أفهامهم. في مقالته في النوم واليقظة.

(١٠) الأبدان التي هي في الغاية القصوى من الحرارة فليس تحتاج إلى رياضة أصلا وتكتفي بالمشي والاستحمام والتمريخ بالدهن تمريخا جيّدا. وقد يوافقهم الاستحمام بعد الطعام. سادسة تدبير الصحّة.

(١١) الشيوخ يحتاجون أن يحرّكوا أبدانهم لأنّ حرارتهم تحتاج إلى الترويح. ولا شيخ واحد يحتاج إلى السكون والدعة الكاملة حتى لا يتحرّك أصلا كما أنّه لا يحتاج إلى رياضة حثيثة لأنّ الرياضة الحثيثة تبرد حرارتهم الضعيفة وتطفئه. خامسة تدبير الصحّة.

(١٢) حدّ الرياضة حركة قوية تغيّر النفس. فمتى تحرّك الإنسان حركة ما اضطرّته أن يتنفّس تنفّسا أزيد عظما وسرعة وتواترا ممّا كان عليه قبل ذلك، فتلك الحركة رياضة لذلك الشخص. ثانية تدبير الصحّة.

(١٣) أفضل أوقات الرياضة هو بعد استكمال انهضام الغذاء الأمسي واستمرائه في البطن والعروق ويكون قد حضر وقت تناول غذاء آخر. ودليل ذلك صفرة البول على حال اعتدال ويقذف جميع ما هو محتبس في المثانة والأمعاء السفلى من الفضل. وبعد ذلك تأمر بالرياضة. ثانية تدبير الصحّة.

---

١ من أفرط في] قال من أفرط في BEOU من أدمن في L || ٣ الرياضة] الرياضات ELOU || ١٢ النفس] التنفس BEOU || ١٣ أزيد عظما] زائدا عظيما G¹ || ١٨ ثانية تدبير الصحّة] في تلك المقالة ELO

(14) Prior to physical exercise you should rub [the patient] and massage his body. Then he should exercise gently and increase [his exertion] until he reaches the optimum level of exercise, that is, as long as his color is healthy and[20] you find him moving quickly, while his movements are even and his sweat is flowing. But as soon as any of these conditions changes, he should stop exercising. *De sanitate tuenda* 2.[21]

(15) After the completion of the exercise, you should pour a generous amount of oil over the body and apply moderate massage while the body is moderately moved and rotated; this massage is called "restorative."[22] Then he should take a bath and wash himself, though he should not stay too long in it, and after the bath he should eat. *De sanitate tuenda* 3.[23]

(16) If a short quartan fever occurs that is not severe, there is no objection if the patient does some of his usual exercises in the days of the abatement [of the fever]. *Ad Glauconem [de methodo medendi].*[24]

This is the end of the eighteenth treatise, by the grace of God, praise be to Him.

(١٤) ينبغي أن تتقدّم وتدلك البدن وتمرخه قبل الرياضة. ثمّ يرتاض برفق و يتدرّج حتّى يصل غاية رياضته وهو كلّ ما حسن لونه وتجده مسارعا إلى الحركة وتجد حركاته متساوية وعرقه يجري. وأوّل ما يتغيّر شيء من هذه الأحوال يمسك عن الرياضة. ثانية تدبير الصحّة.

(١٥) بعد انتهاء الرياضة تغرق البدن بالدهن وتدلكه دلكا معتدلا وهو يتحرّك و يتقلّب حركة معتدلة وهذا هو الاسترداد. ثمّ يدخل الحمّام و يغتسل ولا يطيل فيه و بعد الحمّام يتناول الطعام. ثالثة تدبير الصحّة.

(١٦) إن كانت حمّى الربع القصيرة ولم تكن بالصعبة فلا بأس أن يستعمل صاحبها بعض الرياضة التي قد جرت بها عادته في يومي راحته. أولى أغلوقن.

تمّت المقالة الثامنة عشر وللّه الحمد والمنّة.

٢ حركاته ELOU | حرارته ELOU || ٣ ثانية تدبير الصحّة | في تلك المقالة ELO || ٩ تمّت المقالة الثامنة عشر وللّه الحمد والمنّة om. B | تمّت المقالة الثامنة عشر وللّه الحمد والمنّة وعدد فصولها سبعة عشر فصلا E كملت المقالة وعدد فصولها سبعة عشر فصلا L تمّت المقالة الثامنة عشر والحمد للّه وعدد فصولها سبعة عشر فصلا O تمّت المقالة العاشرة لجيش والحمد للّه عدد فصولها سبعة عشر U

The Nineteenth Treatise

Containing aphorisms concerning bathing[1]

(1) Bathing[2] evacuates only that which is near the skin. That which is deep inside the body, spread in the flesh, is not adequately evacuated by bathing. *In Hippocratis Aphorismos commentarius* 3.[3]

(2) Bathing is beneficial for the other[4] types of dryness, whether [that dryness] comes with cold (as in the case of marasmus), from old age, or with heat (as in the case of hectic fevers that are free from putrefaction). This characteristic of bathing is wonderful in that it is beneficial for both hot and cold dryness, and it likewise makes him thirsty who does not suffer from thirst and quenches the thirst of him who is thirsty. *De marcore.*[5]

(3) Using the baths weakens the faculties [of the body] if it has been a long time since one has eaten and[6] one is very hungry. This also happens as a result of [bathing] in the case of all the other bodily conditions. If one bathes before the digestion of the food, it causes the accumulation of crude chymes in the body. The best time for [bathing] is after the digestion of food, since then it helps pass the food into the organs. *De marcore.*[7]

بسم الله الرحمن الرحيم

ربّ يسّر

المقالة التاسعة عشر

تشتمل على فصول تتعلّق بالحمّام

(١) الحمّام يستفرغ ممّا يلي الجلد فقط. أمّا ما هو في عمق البدن منبثّ في اللحم فليس
يستفرغه الحمّام استفراغا كافيا. في شرحه لثالثة الفصول.

(٢) الحمّام ينفع سائر أصناف اليبس كان مع برودة كالذبول الشيخوخي أو مع حرارة
كحمّيات الدقّ السالمة من عفونة. وهذه الخلّة عجيبة في الحمّام فإنّه ينفع اليبس الحارّ واليبس
البارد وكذلك يحدث العطش لمن ليس به عطش ويقطع العطش عن من به عطش. في مقالته
في الذبول.

(٣) الحمّام إذا استعمل بعد عهد طويل بالطعام وحاجة شديدة إلى الغذاء أوهن القوى
ويعرض ذلك منه في سائر الحالات للبدن. وإن استعمل قبل انهضام الطعام كان سببا لاجتماع
الكيموسات الفجّة في البدن. وأفضل أوقاته بعد انهضام الغذاء فحينئذ يعين على نفوذ الغذاء
إلى الأعضاء. في تلك المقالة.

١ بسم الله الرحمن الرحيم ربّ يسّر [om. BELU بسم الله الرحمن الرحيم O ‖ ٥ البدن] om. G ‖ ٦ كافيا]
شافيا ELO ‖ ٨ الخلّة] الخصلة L ‖ ١٢ الحالات للبدن] حالات البدن BELOU

(4) Bathing is one of the most beneficial things for someone who is to be evacuated of superfluities streaming into his stomach. However, nosebleed and other hemorrhages are strongly stimulated by bathing. And if someone develops syncope because of profuse sweating, bathing is one of the most harmful things for him [to do]. *Ad Glauconem [de methodo medendi]* 1.[8]

[(5)][9]

(6) Bathing in nitrous or sulfurous water and other kinds of water with drying strength dries the body. Frequent bathing in sweet water, especially after eating, moistens the body. *De [morborum] causis et symptomatibus* 2.[10]

(7) One should bathe in drinkable[11] water of[12] a moderate temperature. The most appropriate thing to do if bathing in cold water is to jump into it all at once so that the water reaches all parts of the body at the same time and one does not shiver. *De sanitate tuenda* 3.[13]

(8) After bathing in cold water one has more appetite, better digestion, less thirst, a stronger body in general, and skin that is in the best [possible] condition, that is, harder and firmer. *De sanitate tuenda* 3.[14]

(9) Moderate heat combined with moisture, such as the heat of a bath, has the potential to cool, but the waters should be sweet and drinkable, for these waters cool and moisten the body of him who bathes in them. *In Hippocratis Epidemiarum librum* 6 *commentaria* 5.[15]

(٤) الحمّام من أوفق الأشياء لمن استفراغه من أشياء تنصبّ إلى معدته. وأمّا الرعاف وسائر انفجار الدم فيهيّجه الحمّام تهيّجا شديدا. ومن أصابه أيضا الغشي من كثرة العرق فالحمّام من أضرّ الأشياء له. أولى من أغلوقن.

(٥)

(٦) الاستحمام بالماء الذي تخالطه قوته البورق والكبريت وغيره ممّا قوتة قوته يابسة تجفّف البدن وتيبّسه. والاستحمام الكثير بالماء العذب ولا سيّما بعد الطعام يرطّب البدن. ثانية العلل والأعراض.

(٧) ينبغي أن يكون الاستحمام بالماء المشروب المعتدل في مزاجه. وأولى الأمور في الاستحمام بالماء البارد أن يزجّ نفسه فيه دفعة حتّى يلقى الماء أعضاءه كلّها في زمان واحد ولا تحدث له قشعريرة. ثالثة تدبير الصحّة.

(٨) بعقب الاستحمام بالماء البارد تكثر الشهوة للطعام ويجوّد الاستمراء ويقلّ العطش ويشدّ البدن بأسره ويصير الجلد على أفضل حالاته وذلك أنّه يزيده صلابة واستحصافا. ثالثة تدبير الصحّة.

(٩) الحرارة المعتدلة التي معها رطوبة مثل حرارة الحمّام تبرد بالقوة وينبغي أن تكون المياه عذبة شروبة فإنّ هذه المياه تبرد بدن المستعمل لها وترطّبه. في الخامسة من شرحه لسادسة أبيديميا.

١ من [om. BELO ‏٤ || The enumeration (٥) follows the Hebrew translation by Muntner and the English one by Rosner. The missing aphorism is one allegedly found by Muntner in one of the Arabic manuscripts. ٥ (٦)–(١٣): om. B ‏|| ٨ المشروب [الشروب OU ‏|| ٩ يزجّ [يجز G ‏|| ١٦ أبيديميا [أفيديميا ELO

(10) You should know that there is nothing better than sleep after bathing for concocting that which can be concocted and for dissolving and dispelling the bad humors. *De sanitate tuenda* 4.[16]

(11) Bathing in sweet water is the best thing for people from whose bodies a vaporous superfluity dissolves while they are healthy. If you prevent these and their like from bathing, they develop a fever. Someone who suffers from fever because of firmness[17] of the skin [also] needs bathing. Similarly, someone who suffers from fever because of exposure to the sun should first of all be cooled, and once his fever has abated, let him take a bath. *De methodo medendi* 8.[18]

(12) Bathing is most harmful for those whose bodies contain many raw, crude humors. The same applies to very hot or cold air, because bathing and very hot air dissolve their humors so that they stream from one organ to another and one cannot be sure that they will not stream to the major organs or other eminent internal organs. Very cold air makes the concoction of these humors difficult; they can be cured, however, by drinking wine with hot water because this helps the concoction of the crude humors. *De methodo medendi* 12.[19]

(13) One whose body is emaciated benefits from bathing after meals. But someone who bathes after meals cannot be sure that no obstruction will occur in his liver. If this regimen is continued for a long time, it causes stones in his kidneys. If he has a sensation of heaviness in his right side and in his loins, he should immediately eat capers [*Capparis spinosa*] with vinegar and honey at the beginning of his meal and continue to do so until the [feeling of] heaviness disappears. *De methodo medendi* 14.[20]

(14) If someone suffers from biting humors that irritate the cardia of his stomach, one should hasten, after bathing, to feed him with that which produces good blood. If this is only possible before the bath, he should take such a quantity that does not harm him during bathing. *Mayāmir* 2.[21]

(١٠) قد ينبغي أن تعلم أنّه ليس شيء يبلغ مبلغ النوم بعقب الحمّام في إنضاج ما يتهيّأ إنضاجه وتحليل الأخلاط الرديئة وفشّها. رابعة تدبير الصحّة.

(١١) أجود ما يستعمل أصحاب الأبدان التي يتحلّل منها فضل دخاني في حال صحّته الاستحمام بالماء العذب. وإن أنت منعت هؤلاء وأمثالهم من الاستحمام حمّوا. وكذلك من حمّ من استحصاف يحتاج إلى الحمّام وكذلك من حمّ من التعرّض للشمس تبرّده أوّلا وإذا انحطّت حمّاه أدخله الحمّام. ثامنة الحيلة.

(١٢) الذين في أبدانهم أخلاط نيئة خامة كثيرة فالحمّام أضرّ شيئ لهم. وكذلك الهواء الحارّ جدّا أو البارد جدّا لأنّ الحمّام والهواء الحارّ جدّا تذيب أخلاطهم فتنصبّ من عضو إلى عضو فلا يؤمن انصبابها إلى أعضاء رئيسة أو غيرها من أعضاء باطنة لها شرف. والهواء البارد جدّا يعسر نضجها. وإنّما شفاؤهم بشرب شراب بماء حارّ فإنّ ذلك يعين على نضج الأخلاط الخامة. ثانية عشر الحيلة.

(١٣) من كان بدنه قد نحف يستنفع بالاستحمام بعد الطعام ولكنْ ليس يؤمن من استحمّ بعد الطعام أن يعرض له سدد في كبده. وإذا طال هذا التدبير يولّد له حصى في الكليتين فإذا وجد مسّ الثقل في جانبه الأيمن وفي قطنه فليطعم على المكان الكبر بخلّ وعسل في أوّل طعامه ولا يزال كذلك حتّى يذهب الثقل. آخر الحيلة.

(١٤) إن كانت الأخلاط لذّاعة تلذع فم معدته فينبغي أن يبادر بإطعامه ما يولّد دما محمودا بعد الحمّام. وإن لم يمكن إلّا قبل الحمّام فليكن ما يتناول مقدارا لا يضرّه عند الاستحمام. ثانية الميامر

(15) Bathing in sweet water is beneficial for the organs of the voice and the other organs affected by tiredness. Those[22] who [professionally] use a high voice frequently enter the bathhouse and have a bath and eat foods that do not bite but instead have a slackening effect. *Mayāmir* 7.[23]

(16) Bathing is most beneficial for those [suffering from] an opthalmia if it is thoroughly ripe and the body is clean, for the pain subsides immediately and the flow of moisture that streams towards the eye stops and the humors become balanced and mixed. *De methodo medendi* 13.[24]

(17) For those suffering from an affection of the spleen, poultices should be applied to the spleen after two hours of the day [have passed] until the ninth hour. The patient should enter the bathhouse while the poultice [still] adheres to him. When it becomes loose and then falls off in the bathhouse, let[25] him go into the bathing basin. *Mayāmir* 9.[26]

(18) It is best for someone who[27] cannot enter the bathhouse after exercise in the beginning of the day to eat bread only in a quantity that his stomach can digest prior to the time that he takes a bath. *De sanitate tuenda* 6.[28]

(19) If headaches originate from a hot dyscrasia, baths in drinkable water should be administered frequently because that disperses the hot vapors originating in the head and completely changes the temperament of the body for the better. If the head is very warm and burning, the best thing [to do] in the summer is to rub the head with oil of roses prepared with omphacine[29] oil. *De sanitate tuenda* 6.[30]

(20) Cold and moist bodies [are prone to] deterioration; they quickly suffer from diseases [originating] from the streaming of superfluities. Those who suffer from such a condition benefit from abstention from bathing, from physical exercise, and from [adherence to] a thinning regimen. *De sanitate tuenda* 6.[31]

(١٥) ممّا ينفع آلات الصوت وسائر الأعضاء التي يصيبها الإعياء الاستحمام بالماء العذب. والذين يستعملون أصواتهم مرتفعة يستعملون دخول الحمّام والاستحمام فيه كثيرا ويأكلون من الطعام ما كان لا يلذع بل يرخي. سابعة الميامر.

(١٦) إذا نضج الرمد واستحكم نضجه وكان البدن نقيًا فالحمّام من أنفع الأشياء لهؤلاء وذلك أنّ الوجع يسكن من ساعته وينقطع به سيلان الرطوبة التي كانت تسيل إلى العين وتعتدل الأخلاط وتمتزج. ثالثة عشر الحيلة.

(١٧) أضمدة المطحولين تجعل على الطحال من بعد ساعتين من نهار إلى آخر التاسعة. ويدخل المريض الحمّام والضماد لاصق به فإذا استرخى الضماد وسقط في الحمّام بعد ذلك ادخله الأبزن. تاسعة الميامر.

(١٨) أصلح الأحوال لمن لا يمكنه دخول الحمّام بعد الرياضة أوّل النهار أن يتناول من الخبز وحده بمقدار ما تهضمه معدته قبل وقت دخوله الحمّام. سادسة تدبير الصحة.

(١٩) إن كانت علل الرأس من سوء مزاج حارّ فينبغي استعمال الحمّام كثيرا بالماء المشروب. فإنّ هذا يفشّ البخارات الحارّة المتولّدة في الرأس ويغيّر مزاج البدن بأسره إلى ما هو أجود. وإن كان الرأس شديد الحرارة والتوقّد فالأصلح أن يدهن في الصيف بدهن الورد المتّخذ بزيت الإنفاق. سادسة تدبير الصحّة.

(٢٠) الأبدان الباردة الرطبة رديئة تسرع إليها الأمراض التي من سيلان الفضول. وممّا ينتفع به أصحاب هذه الحال الإمساك عن الاستحمام وعن الرياضات وتلطيف التدبير. سادسة تدبير الصحّة.

---

١ الاستحمام] الحمّام G || ٦ وتمتزج] وتتميّز EL || ١٢ سوء مزاج] بخار L || الحمّام] الاستحمام G¹ || ١٦ رديئة] الرديئة BEL || ١٧ الرياضات] الرياضة BELOU

(21) For him in whose body vaporous superfluities originate, bathing is appropriate, even twice a day and especially in the summer. But if someone with a cold and moist temperament abandons bathing, it is not harmful for him. A cold and dry temperament needs bathing, as is the case with the elderly. Superfluities increase in the bodies of those who have a hot and moist temperament; the application of bathing before the evacuation [of these superfluities] is dangerous, but after the evacuation it is beneficial. *De sanitate tuenda* 5.[32]

(22) Someone whose body is full of raw, crude humors should not take a bath, for bathing prompts those humors to exit [and] they quickly obstruct the narrow channels. *De sanitate tuenda* 4.[33]

(23) He says concerning the regimen of those suffering from quartan fever in its initial phase: As for massage, walking, bathing, and their other usual activities, one should not withhold these from them completely. But if they can completely abstain from bathing and be satisfied with massage only, it is most beneficial to them. *Ad Glauconem de methodo medendi* 1.[34]

(24) A thick humor dissolves and becomes thinner by drinking pure wine and by taking a bath immediately thereafter. *In Hippocratis Aphorismos commentarius* 7.[35]

(25) Hippocrates says in the third [book] of his *[Regimen] on acute diseases* and Galen in his commentary thereon that those who suffer from pleurisy, pneumonia, and acute fevers benefit from bathing. *In Hippocratis De acutorum morborum [victu] commentarius* 3.[36]

(26) Says Moses: That sufferers from fever benefit from bathing after the concoction [of their humors] is a subject raised in several sections of Galen's books.[37] As for the statement of both [Hippocrates and Galen] that bathing is beneficial for pleurisy and pneumonia, it seems to me that they are referring to those who suffer from pain in the side or in the lungs because of a dyscrasia or because of thick or biting humors but without inflammation or fever. These are the patients who benefit from bathing.

(٢١) من كانت تتولّد فيه فضول دخانية فالذي يصلح له الاستحمام ولو مرّتين كلّ يوم ولا سيّما في الصيف. وأمّا من كان مزاجه باردا رطبا فإنّه إن ترك الحمّام لا يضرّه ذلك. والمزاج البارد اليابس يحتاج إلى الحمّام كالشيوخ. وأمّا أصحاب والمزاج الحارّ الرطب فإنّ الفضول تكثر في أبدانهم واستعمال الحمّام فيهم قبل الاستفراغ خطر وبعد الاستفراغ نافع.

٥ خامسة تدبير الصحّة.

(٢٢) من كان بدنه مملوءًا أخلاطا نيئة فجّة فلا ينبغي أن يدخل الحمّام فإنّ الحمّام يستدعي تلك الأخلاط للخروج فتسبق وتسدّ المجاري الضيّقة. رابعة تدبير الصحّة.

(٢٣) قال في تدبير أصحاب حمّى الربع في أوّلها: أمّا الدلك والمشي ودخول الحمّام وسائر ما جرت به عادتهم فلا تمنعهم منه المنع التامّ إلّا أنّهم إن قدروا على الإمساك أصلا عن الاستحمام واقتصروا على الدلك وحده كان ذلك أبلغ لهم في الانتفاع. أولى أغلوقن.

١٠

(٢٤) الخلط الغليظ يذوب ويرقّ بشرب الشراب الصرف واستعمال الحمّام في عقب شربه. في شرحه لسابعة الفصول.

(٢٥) يقول بقراط في ثالثة الأمراض الحادّة وجالينوس في شرحه لذلك الكلام إنّ أصحاب ذات الجنب وذات الرئة وأصحاب الحمّيات الحادّة ينتفعون بالحمّام.

(٢٦) قال موسى: أمّا أنّ أصحاب الحمّيات ينتفعون بالحمّام بعد النضج فسيأتيك في ذلك ١٥ فصول من كلام جالينوس. وأمّا قولهما في نفع الحمّام لصاحب ذات الجنب وذات الرئة فالذي يبدو إليّ أنّهما يريدان بذلك من به وجع جنب أو وجع رئة من سوء مزاج أو من أخلاط غليظة أو لذّاعة من غير ورم ولا حمّى وهذا هو الذي يستنفع بالحمّام.

١ ولو | om. O وهي | EL ٦ فإنّ | لأنّ BELOU ‖ om. G ‖ ٨ أصحاب | om. G ‖ ١٣ بقراط | أبقراط BELOU ‖ ١٥ في | من BEOU

(27) Bathing is beneficial for someone suffering from diarrhea because it attracts the [superfluous] matters to the skin.[38] But someone whose body is full or who is constipated should not take a bath.[39] *In Hippocratis De acutorum morborum [victu] commentarius* 3.

(28) Someone suffering from a nosebleed or nausea or bilious super-fluities in his stomach should not take a bath. If he does so, he ruins his strength and brings about syncope. Similarly, someone whose strength is weak should not bathe. *In Hippocratis De acutorum morborum [victu] commentarius* 3.[40]

(29) In the case of fevers, one should bathe after the concoction [of the humors] so that it helps the completion [of the concoction] and dis-solves [the humors]. One should be wary of bathing before the concoc-tion and, in general, be very cautious in the case of fevers caused by salty putrid phlegm because the phlegm cannot be dissolved through the skin [in the way that] bile can be dissolved, nor can its heat be extinguished or suppressed. *In Hippocratis De acutorum morborum [victu] commentarius* 3.[41]

(30) One should thoroughly dry one's head after bathing so that no moisture remains on it, not even a little quantity, because that remain-ing quantity cools the brain [and thus harms it]. *In Hippocratis De acuto-rum morborum [victu] commentarius* 3.[42]

(31) During chymous fevers, taking a bath after the chymes have been concocted has a healing effect. It is appropriate at all times for hectic fever. There is no need to be afraid of bathing in the case of these fevers unless one's strength is very weak or the hectic fever comes with a putrefying fever. But do not let the patient take a bath until the chymes are concocted. *De marcore.*[43]

(32) All patients with ephemeral fever should take a bath, except for those to whom this fever occurred because of firmness of the skin or because of a swelling of the glands in the groin or armpit. But if you tell these patients to stay in the air of the bathhouse for a long time, it will not harm them at all. All other patients affected by [this fever], if it occurred to them from causes other than the two mentioned, should stay

(٢٧) الاستحمام ينفع من به إسهال لأنّه يجذب الموادّ إلى الجلد. ولا ينبغي أن يدخل الحمّام مَن بدنه ممتلئ ولا من في بطنه معتقل. في شرحه لثالثة الأمراض الحادّة.

(٢٨) لا يستعمل الحمّام من به رعاف أو غثي أو من في معدته مرار. وإن فعل أسقط القوة وأحدث الغثي. وكذلك يجتنب الاستحمام من قوته ضعيفة. في شرحه لثالثة الأمراض الحادّة.

(٢٩) إنّما ينبغي أن يستعمل الاستحمام في الحمّيات بعد النضج ليعين على تمامه ويحلّل. وينبغي أن يحذر قبل النضج ويحذر بالجملة في ما كان من الحمّيات عن بلغم مالح عفن لأنّ البلغم لا يتحلّل من الجلد كما يتحلّل المرار وحرارته لا تطفأ ولا تخمد. في شرحه لثالثة الأمراض الحادّة.

(٣٠) ينبغي أن ينشّف الرأس بعد الاستحمام تنشيفا مستقصيا حتّى لا يبقى عليه شيء من الرطوبة ولو قلّ لأنّ ذلك الباقي يبرد فيتأذّى الدماغ. في شرحه لثالثة الأمراض الحادّة.

(٣١) استعمال الحمّام في حمّيات الكيموسات بعد نضج الكيموسات يشفي وهو في كلّ الأوقات يلائم حمّى الدقّ ولا خوف منه في هذه الحمّيات إلّا أن تكون القوة ضعيفة جدًّا أو تقترن بحمّى الدقّ حمّى عفنية. ولا تدخله الحمّام حتّى تنضج الكيموسات. في مقالته في الذبول.

(٣٢) أصحاب حمّى يوم جميعهم ينبغي أن يدخلوا الحمّام إلّا من عرضت له هذه الحمّى بسبب استحصاف الجلد أو بسبب ورم الغدد التي في الأربية والإبط. فإن أمرته أن يطيل اللبث في هواء الحمّام لم يضرّه ذلك شيئا. وأمّا سائر من عرضت له من غير هذين السببين

in the air of the bathhouse for a short time only, but are allowed to stay in the water as long as they wish. *Ad Glauconem [de methodo medendi]* 1.[44]

(33) Those suffering from pure tertian fever are allowed to bathe in sweet, drinkable hot water since it extracts and evacuates some of the bile and is extremely beneficial because of its quality. For bathing in this water moistens, cools, and strengthens the body. Your intention in letting someone suffering from this fever have a bath should be to moisten and wet his body. *Ad Glauconem [de methodo medendi]* 1.[45]

(34) People suffering from marasmus and all those in whom dryness prevails do not need the hot air in the bathhouse, but rather the extremely temperate water of the bathing basin. Big bathing basins are better than small ones for this illness. The patient should remain in the water for a very long time. The water should be extremely temperate and pleasant so[46] that it encourages the nature [of the patient] to spread, open, and expand in every direction to meet with that which gives it pleasure to enjoy. It is sufficient when [his body] is moderately heated in the bath.[47] Then, after the bathing, you should massage him with oil so that the pores of his skin are closed, the acquired moisture spreads within the body, and he is not harmed by the air. *De methodo [medendi]* 7.[48]

(35) If someone of those who have vaporous superfluities develops a fever from becoming chilled, he should take a bath, unless the fever is accompanied by a catarrh or rheum. But do not let him take a bath when the catarrh or rheum is not ripe. If someone has a fever because[49] he has been burned by the sun, he should take a bath even if he has a catarrh or rheum. After the bath, pour cooled rose oil over his head in the same way as you did before the bath. *De methodo [medendi]* 8.[50]

(36) For all patients with hectic fever, and especially for those suffering from marasmus, taking a cold water bath without [first] bathing [in hot water] is dangerous, because prior bathing [in hot water] warms the body, prepares it, and makes it ready for bathing in cold water. *De methodo [medendi]* 10.[51]

Once signs of concoction [of the humors] have appeared, taking a bath is beneficial for someone whose fever is only light and whose faculties are not strong. *De methodo [medendi]* 11.[52]

فجميعهم يقلّلون اللبث في هواء الحمّام و يؤذن لهم في الماء ما أحبّوا. في الأولى من أغلوقن.

(٣٣) أصحاب حمّى الغبّ الخالصة يؤذن لهم بالاستحمام بالماء الحارّ العذب المشروب فإنّه يستخرج و يستفرغ أشياء من المرار و ينفع بكيفيته منفعة عظيمة. وذلك أنّ الاستحمام بهذا الماء يرطّب البدن ويبرده ويقوّيه. وينبغي أن يكون غرضك في إدخال صاحب هذه الحمّى الحمّام أن تبلّ بدنه وترطّبه. أولى أغلوقن.

٥

(٣٤) المذبولون وكلّ من غلب عليه اليبس فليس يحتاج من الحمّام إلى الهواء الحارّ بل إلى ماء الأبزن الذي في غاية الاعتدال. والأبزنات الكبار أفضل من الصغار لهذا المرض. وينبغي أن يلبث في الماء زمانا أطول وكيفية الماء المعتدلة في الغاية تستلذّ فهي لذلك تحرّك الطبيعة للانبساط والتفتيح والتمدّد إلى كلّ ناحية لتلقى الشيء السارّ لها بما تستلذّ منه. وحسبك منه أن يسخن سخونة معتدلة في الحمّام. ثمّ تمسحه بالدهن بعد الاستحمام لتسدّ مسامّ الجلد منه لينبثّ ما حصل من الرطوبة داخل الجسم ولأن لا تباده من الهواء مضرّة. سابعة الحيلة.

١٠

(٣٥) من حمّ من أصحاب الفضل الدخاني من برد أصابه فينبغي أن يدخل الحمّام إلّا أن كان حمّى مع نزلة أو زكام. فلا تدخله الحمّام دون أن تنضج نزلته أو زكامه. فأمّا من حمّ من قبل شمس أحرقته فينبغي أن يدخل الحمّام و إن كان به زكام أو نزلة وبعد الحمّام تصبّ على رؤسهم دهن الورد المبرّد كما فعلت قبل الحمّام. ثامنة الحيلة.

١٥

(٣٦) جميع أصحاب حمّى الدقّ وبخاصّة من وقع إلى الذبول دخوله الماء البارد من غير حمّام خطر لأنّ الحمّام يتقدّم ويسخن البدن ويهيّئه ويعدّه للاستحمام بالماء البارد. عاشرة الحيلة. الحمّام نافع لمن كانت حمّاه يسيرة وقواه ليست بالقوية بعد ظهور علامات النضج. حادثة عشر الحيلة.

---

١ لهم في الماء ما أحبّوا] له في الماء ما أحبّ L || ٦ المذبولون] المذبولين BELOU | يحتاج] إليه add. G¹ ||
١١ تباده] تناله E تدنوه L ابتداه B | سابعة] سادسة G || ١٧ ويهيّئه] ويهيجه L

(37) In the case of all fevers, one should pay attention to three things concerning bathing in the bathhouse: [first], that the patient is not affected by a shivering fit when he takes a bath; second, that none of the vital organs is weak; and third, that the primary vessels are not congested by a large quantity of crude humors. *De methodo [medendi]* 11.[53]

For all intermittent fevers, the best time to take a bath, if one is allowed to do so, is when the heat of the fever begins to dissolve, for then the bath immediately prepares the body and makes it fit to be nourished. But in the case of these fevers, one should always beware of going into a cold-water basin. *De methodo [medendi]* 11.[54]

(38) For some people, it is most appropriate to take some food prior to bathing. But for everyone whose temperament is extremely hot and dry it is fitting to bathe after the meal. *De sanitate tuenda* 6.[55]

(39) You should look into the matter of everyone who seems to you to be bathing after eating. If you notice someone experiencing any pain or heaviness or tension in the region of the liver, do not let [that person] with such conditions bathe after meals. If he perceives any such [condition], hasten to open the obstruction of his liver and let him always abstain from thick foods. *De sanitate tuenda* 6.[56]

This is the end of the nineteenth treatise by the grace of God, praise be to Him.

(٣٧) الاستحمام في الحمّام في الحمّيات كلّها ينبغي أن يقصد فيه ثلاثة أغراض: أحدها أن لا يحدث نافض الاقشعرار عند دخوله والثاني أن لا يكون واحد من الأعضاء النفيسة ضعيفا والثالث أن لا يكون في العروق الأوّل من الأخلاط النيئة مقدار كثير محتقن. حادية عشر الحيلة. أصلح الأوقات لدخول الحمّام في جميع الحمّيات المقلعة إذا جاز دخوله هو وقت أن تبتدئ حرارة الحمّى تتحلّل فإنّ الحمّام حينئذ يهيّئ البدن من ساعته و يصلحه للغذاء. وتحذر أبدا في هذه الحمّيات دخول حوض الماء البارد. حادية عشر الحيلة.

(٣٨) الأصلح لبعض الناس أن يتناول شيئا من الطعام قبل الحمّام. وكلّ من مزاجه حارّ يابس في الغاية القصوى قد يوافقه الاستحمام بعد الطعام. سادسة تدبير الصحّة.

(٣٩) كلّ من يبدو لك أنّه يحمّ بعد الطعام فينبغي أن تفتقد أمره. فإن رأيت أنّه يجد في موضع الكبد شيئا من الوجع أو ثقلا أو تمدّدا فجنّب كلّ من هيئاته هكذا الاستحمام بعد الطعام. فإن وجدوا شيئا من ذلك فبادر لتفتيح سدد كبدهم وجنّبهم أبدا الأطعمة الغليظة. سادسة تدبير الصحّة.

تمّت المقالة التاسعة عشر وللّه الحمد والمنّة.

١ أحدها] أوّلها L ‖ ٣ حادية عشر الحيلة] في تلك المقالة ELO ‖ ٦ أبدا] أيضا L ‖ حادية عشر الحيلة] في تلك المقالة ELO ‖ ٩ أنّه يحمّ] أنّك تحمّه ELO أن يجد تخمة B أنّه تحمّه U ‖ رأيت أنّه] رأيته BELOU ‖ ١٠ موضع] om. G ‖ ١٣ تمّت المقالة التاسعة عشر وللّه الحمد والمنّة] om. B تمّت المقالة التاسعة عشر والحمد للّه والمنّة كثير كما هو أعلم E تمّت المقالة وعدد فصولها أربعون فصلا L تمّت المقالة التاسعة عشر والحمد للّه وعدد فصولها أربعون فصلا O تمّت المقالة الحادي عشر عدد فصولها تسعة وثلاثين U

In the name of God,
the Merciful, the Compassionate.
O Lord, make [our task] easy.

The Twentieth Treatise

Containing aphorisms concerning
foods, beverages, and their consumption

(1) Our first specific goal in the consumption of foods is that the food will be well digested. Our second goal thereafter is that[1] the chyme produced therefrom will be beneficial, that is, that it fits all the other organs. *De bonis [malisque] sucis.*[2]

(2) The knowledge of the powers of the [different] foods is nearly the most useful kind of knowledge in the field of medicine, since there is a constant and never-ending need for food, during both health and sickness. *De alimentorum facultatibus* 1.[3]

(3) Helpful to repel the harm caused by bad foodstuff is [the following]: the consumption of only a small amount of it, habit, bodily activity, and a long sleep after its consumption. *De alimentorum facultatibus* 1.[4]

بسم الله الرحمن الرحيم

ربّ يسّر

المقالة العشرون

تشتمل على فصول تتعلّق

بالأغذية والمياه وتناولها ٥

(١) غرضنا الأوّل الخاصّ في استعمال الأغذية هو أن ينهضم الغذاء انهضاما حسنا

وغرضنا الثاني بعد هذا هو أن يكون الكيموس المتولّد منه محمودا، أعني أنّه يلائم سائر

الأعضاء. في مقالته في جودة الكيموس.

(٢) العلم بقوى الأغذية قريب من أن يكون أنفع علوم الطبّ إذ كانت الحاجة إلى

الغذاء دائما أبدا في وقت الصحّة ووقت المرض. أوّل الأغذية. ١٠

(٣) يعين على دفع مضرّة الأغذية الرديئة نزارة ما يستعمل منها والعادة والرياضة وطول

النوم بعد تناولها. أوّل الأغذية.

---

١ بسم الله الرحمن الرحيم ربّ يسّر | om. BELU ‖ ٣ المقالة العشرون | بالماء والغذاء المقالة الحادي عشر
لجبيس U | العشرون B | العشقنينة B ‖ ١١ الرديئة | L¹ | نزارة | شرّ O | ١٢ أوّل الأغذية | في تلك المقالة ELO

(4) For any individual person, the digestion of the food he eats can be easy or difficult, either through[5] its specific substance and nature, or[6] through the occurrence of a symptom. *De alimentorum facultatibus* 2.[7]

(5) We as physicians focus especially on the benefit that foods should provide, not on the pleasure to be derived from them. But since some foods are distasteful and their distastefulness hinders their digestion, the physician should make efforts to season such food so that it can be well digested. However, cooks [usually] season food [to such a degree] that it contributes to a bad digestion. *De alimentorum facultatibus* 2.[8]

(6) Soft food is easier and faster to digest in the stomach, to turn into blood in the liver and the vessels, and to be absorbed into every single organ that is nourished by it. But harder food is more difficult [to digest] and more slow to undergo all [these processes].[9] *De alimentorum facultatibus* 3.[10]

(7) When we are hungry we should not greedily stuff ourselves with food like a dog, and when we are thirsty we should not enjoy a cold drink to the same degree as someone whose body is inflamed with[11] continuous fever and who consequently finishes the whole cup out of greed. We should restrain ourselves from stretching out our hands to all that is presented to us or to something sweet and the like, of those things that gluttons take. *De propriorum animi cuiuslibet affectuum dignotione [et curatione].*[12]

(8) Convalescents and weak people should be given stronger food in the evening. But since they cannot digest the food [properly], we should feed them little by little, at various times, and we should let them drink little by little, in such a quantity that their distress is alleviated and their food does not float. *De methodo [medendi]* 7.[13]

(٤) كلّ واحد من الناس يسهل أو يعسر عليه استمراء ما يتناوله من الأغذية إمّا لخصوصية في نفس الجوهر والطبع وإمّا لعارض يعرض. ثانية الأغذية.

(٥) نحن معشر الأطبّاء إنّما نقصد في الأطعمة إلى الانتفاع بها لا إلى التلذّذ. ولمّا كانت أفراد من الأطعمة كريهة وكانت كراهتها تعوقها عن الاستمراء وجب على الطبيب أن يحتال ليطيب ما كان كذلك حتّى يحسن استمراءه. أمّا الطبّاخون فيقصدون تطييب الطعام ولو بما يعين على فساد الاستمراء. ثانية الأغذية.

(٦) الغذاء اللّين أسهل وأسرع قبولا للانهضام في المعدة والاستحالة إلى الدم في الكبد وفي العروق وللتشبّه بكلّ واحد من الأعضاء المغتذية. والأصلب أعسر قبولا لجميع ذلك وأبطأ فيه. ثالثة الأغذية.

(٧) ليس ينبغي لنا بسبب الجوع أن نمتلئ من الطعام امتلاء رغبة كالكلاب ولا بسبب العطش أن نستلذّ الشربة الباردة بمنزلة من قد التهب بدنه بحمّى دائمة فيشرب جميع ما في الكأس بالرغبة. ونتوقّى أكثر من أن نمدّ أيدينا إلى جميع ما يتقدّم لنا ولا إلى الحلو وغيرها ممّا يتّخذه أهل الشره. في مقالته في تعرّف الإنسان عيوب نفسه.

(٨) الناقهون والضعفاء يجعل غذاؤهم بالليل أقوى ولكونهم لا يقدرون على استمراء الطعام نغذوهم شيئا بعد شيء في مرار شتّى ونسقيهم قليلا قليلا بمقدار ما يسكن أذاءهم ولا يطفو طعامهم. سابعة الحيلة.

٥

١٠

١٥

٢ والطبع [om. ELO | ٥ ليطيب [لتطييب BELOU | ٦ ثانية الأغذية [في تلك المقالة ELO || ٧ والاستحالة [وللاستحالة ELOU | ١١ نستلذّ [نستمّ ELO | دائمة [دفعة BELOU | ١٢ بالرغبة [كالجربة ELO || ١٥ بمقدار [بقدر BELOU

(9) If you want to feed convalescents and all those who are weak, you should make it your first aim that the quantity [of food] such a person takes does not overburden him. Your second aim should be that he digest [his food] rapidly, and your third aim should be that it pass quickly [through the bowels]. If you feed them meat of cattle, slaughter [the animal] one day[14] before they are to eat it when it is winter, for the meat that sits overnight is more rapidly digested. But when it is summer, it is enough that the meat be from an animal that has been slaughtered in the morning and is consumed after sunset. *De methodo [medendi]* 7.[15]

(10) Putrid foods and beverages produce corruption similar to that produced by fatal poisons. *In Hippocratis De [aeris] aquis [locis] commentarius* 2.[16]

(11) Food can become beneficial or harmful in its inherent healing powers [for our bodies]. But regarding the nutritional aspect, it is always beneficial for our bodies in all bodily conditions. *In Hippocratis De alimento commentarius* 2.[17]

(12) When [its] strength is weak, [the body] is unable to digest a large [quantity of] food even when its quality is good. Therefore, you should always measure the quantity of food according to the strength or weakness[18] of the body and choose the quality of the food according to the temperament of the body. *In Hippocratis De alimento commentarius* 4.[19]

(13) Some foods soften the stools and relieve the bowels in that they have medicinal powers mixed with them, similar to the powers of scammony [*Convolvulus scammonia*],[20] pulp of colocynth [*Citrullus colocynthis*], and hellebore [*Helleborus* spp.], for these foods have[21] the nature both of food and of medicine. But foods do not fall under the definition of medicines when they do not have any[22] of these influences on the body and do not do anything else but nourish it. There are very few foods of this sort, but[23] those that exist are merely nourishing. *De alimentorum facultatibus* 1.[24]

(٩) الناقهون وكلّ ضعيف تريد أن تغذوه فأوّل ما تجعل غرضك في مقدار ما يتناوله حتّى لا يثقل عليه والثانية سرعة انهضامه والثالثة سرعة انحداره. وإن أطعمتهم لحم المواشي فاذبح لهم قبل أكله بليلة في زمان الشتاء فإنّ اللحم البائت أسرع انهضاما. وإن كان الزمان صيفا فحسبك أن يكون لحم حيوان ذبح باكرا ويؤكل بعد مغيب الشمس. سابعة الحيلة.

٥

(١٠) الأطعمة والأشربة العفنة تولّد فسادا مثل ما تولّد السموم القاتلة. في شرحه للثانية من المياه.

(١١) الغذاء يصير نافعا أو ضارّا بالقوى الدوائية التي فيه. فأمّا من جهة الغذائية فإنّه نافع لأبداننا دائما على كلّ حال من أحوال البدن. في شرحه لثانية الغذاء.

(١٢) القوة الضعيفة لا تقدر على هضم الغذاء الكثير وإن كان جيّدا ولذلك ينبغي أن

١٠

تقدّر كمّية الغذاء أبدا بحسب قوة البدن وضعفه وتختار كيفيته بحسب مزاج البدن. في شرحه لرابعة الغذاء.

(١٣) بعض الأغذية تلين الطبيعة وتطلق البطن من طريق أنّه تخالطه قوى من قوى الأدوية شبيهة بقوة السقمونيا وشحم الحنظل والخربق. وهذه مركّبة مؤلّفة من طبيعة الغذاء وطبيعة الدواء. وإنّما تكون الأغذية خارجة عن حدّ الأدوية متى لم تؤثّر في البدن شيئا من هذه الآثار ولم تعمل شيئا سوى أن تغذوه. وقلّما يوجد من الأغذية على هذه الصفة والذي

١٥

يوجد كذلك هو الغذاء المحض. أولى الأغذية.

٢ سرعة] G¹ || ٣ فاذبح] فتذبح BELOU || ٤ سابعة الحيلة] في تلك المقالة ELO || ٥ الأطعمة . . . القاتلة] وذلك أنّه ليس من أدنا ذهن إلا وهو يعلم أنّ الأطعمة والأشربة العفنة تولّد فسادا مثل ما يتولّد من السموم القتّالة C | القاتلة] القتّالة ELOU

(14) It is impossible for the humor originating from the watermelon [*Citrullus lanatus* var. *lanatus*] to become thick and earth-like, even when it is well digested, just as the humor originating from lentils [*Lens esculenta*] or from beef cannot become watery and moist. Similarly, whenever someone who eats cucumbers [*Cucumis sativus*] does not pay attention to the quantity he eats because he relies on his good digestion, a cold, thick humor collects in his vessels that cannot easily be converted into blood, even if [the cucumbers] are well digested. This[25] is the main thing for the preservation of health and the healing of diseases. *De alimentorum facultatibus* 2.[26]

(15) The dough of bran bread needs only a small amount of yeast, light kneading, and a short time in the oven.[27] But for extremely pure[28] bread the opposite is needed. *De alimentorum facultatibus* 1.[29]

(16) The most beneficial and appropriate bread for[30] someone who does not engage in physical exercise and for the elderly is bread that has been properly baked[31] in an oven and that contains a lot of yeast. But[32] completely unleavened bread is not appropriate for anyone. *De alimentorum facultatibus* 1.[33]

(17) Starch is near in power to washed[34] bread inasmuch[35] as it provides only a little nourishment to the body and does not heat, just as washed bread does not heat, although all the other kinds of bread do heat. *De alimentorum facultatibus* 1.[36]

(18) Our nature prevails over almost all kinds of meat and changes and transforms them and turns them into beneficial blood. But of radishes [*Raphanus sativus* and var.] and beets [*Beta vulgaris*] and the like, only a small part can be changed and transformed, and that only with some trouble and much labor—and [furthermore], that small [part] is not beneficial blood, and the remainder exits with the superfluities. *De naturalibus facultatibus* 1.[37]

(19) The best meat of land animals is pork; then comes the meat of kids and then that of calves. The meat of lambs is moist, sticky, and slimy. As for the meat of the other land animals, I recommend that anyone who cares about keeping his humors in a healthy condition avoid eating it. *De bonis malisque sucis.*[38]

(١٤) ليس يمكن أن يكون الخلط المتولّد من البطّيخ غليظا أرضيا ولو انهضم انهضاما جيّدا كما أنّه لا يتولّد من العدس ولا من لحم البقر خلط مائي رطب. وأكل القثّاء وإن استمراءه استمراء حسنا متى أهمل أمره وأتّكل على جودة هضمه اجتمع في عروقه خلط بارد غليظ لا يستحيل إلى الدم إلّا بعسر. وهذا ملاك الأمر في تدبير الصحّة وشفاء الأمراض. ثانية الأغذية.

(١٥) عجين الخبز الخشكار قد يكتفي بالتخمير اليسير والعجين الضعيف واللبث القليل في النار. والخبز النقي غاية النقاء بعكس ذلك. أولى الأغذية.

(١٦) الأنفع والأوفق لمن لا يقرب الرياضة وللشيوخ ما كان من الخبز قد نضج في التنّور على ما ينبغي وكان فيه من الخمير مقدار كثير. وأمّا الخبز الفطير على وجهه فغير موافق لأحد من الناس. أولى الأغذية.

(١٧) النشاء قوته قريبة من قوة الخبز المغسول من قبل أنّه يغذو البدن غذاء يسيرا ولا يسخن كما لا يسخن الخبز المغسول على أنّ جميع أنواع الخبز تسخن. أولى الأغذية.

(١٨) طبيعتنا تستولي على اللحمان عن آخرها إلّا الشاذّ فتحيلها وتغيّرها وتصير منها دما محمودا. وأمّا الفجل والسلق ونحوها فبكدّ ما يستحيل ويتغيّر منها الشيء اليسير وبالعمل الكثير. وذلك اليسير ليس بدم محمود وبقيتها تخرج مع الفضول. في الأولى من القوى الطبيعية.

(١٩) أفضل اللحمان من الحيوان المشي لحم الخنزير والذي يتلوه لحم الجداء وبعده لحم العجول. وأمّا لحم الحملان فهو رطب لزج مخاطي. وأمّا سائر لحمان الحيوان المشي فإنّي آمر من كان يعني بحسن حال الكيموس أن يمتنع من أكله. في مقالته في جودة الكيموس ورداءته.

***

٩ أوّل الأغذية] في تلك المقالة ELO || ١١ أوّل الأغذية] في تلك المقالة ELO || ١٦ العجول] العجاجيل BELOU | سائر لحمان الحيوان] لحم سائر الحيوان E | لحمان] لحوم E

(20) Because of its lightness, the meat of birds produces a large quantity of bile if it encounters increased heat from the body. *In Hippocratis Epidemiarum librum 6 commentaria* 6.[39]

(21) Roasted [meat] strengthens the body more than boiled [meat]. After this [comes] braised [meat], for braised [meat] strengthens more than any other form of cooked [meat]. *In Hippocratis De alimento commentarius* 4.[40]

(22) The nourishment that the body receives from all meat that is roasted or baked is drier, whereas the nourishment of all meat that is boiled in water is more moist. All meat boiled in a pot and seasoned with spices and condiments falls between these. *De alimentorum facultatibus* 3.[41]

Testicles taste[42] bad and produce bad [humors]. This statement applies only to the testicles of land animals, for the testicles of fatted cocks are delicious and provide good nourishment. [The consumption of] any brain is harmful for the stomach. *De alimentorum facultatibus* 3.[43]

(23) The food[44] provided by wild animals—that it, those that live[45] in the mountains and deserts—does not contain any superfluities. For this reason, [the nutrition] that the [human] body receives from the meat of wild animals is necessarily stronger and better than that which it receives from the meat of domestic animals. *De alimentorum facultatibus* 3.[46]

(24) Wine mixed with an equal amount of water heats the whole body and rapidly moves to all its limbs. It ameliorates and improves the humors of the body by balancing their temperament and by evacuating bad humors. *In Hippocratis Aphorismos commentarius* 7.[47]

(٢٠) لحم الطير لخفّته إذا صادف من البدن حرارة زائدة ولّد مرارا كثيرا. في السادسة
من شرحه لسادسة أبيدِيما.

(٢١) الشواء يقوّي الأبدان أكثر من المطبوخ وبعده المسلوق. والمسلوق يقوّي أكثر من
غيره من أنواع الطبيخ. في الرابعة من شرحه للغذاء.

(٢٢) كلّ لحم يؤكل مشويا أو مطجّنا فالذي ينال البدن منه غذاء أزيد يبسا. وكلّ لحم
يسلق بالماء فغذاؤه أزيد رطوبة. وكلّ لحم يطبخ في قدر ويطيّب بالأبازير والتوابل فحاله
وسط بين الحالين. ثالثة الأغذية.

الخصيتان فيهما زهومة مع رداءة ما يتولّد منها. وقولي هذا في خصى الحيوانات المواشي
لأنّ خصى الديوك المسمّنة لذيذة جدّا وغذاؤها غذاء جيّد. وكلّ دماغ ضارّ للمعدة أيّ
الأدمغة كان. ثالثة الأغذية.

(٢٣) الحيوانات البرّية وهي التي ترعى في الجبال والبراري الغذاء المتولّد منها ليس فيه
فضول. فيجب من هذا الوجه ضرورة أن يكون ما يناله البدن من لحوم الحيوانات البرّية
أكثر ممّا يناله من لحوم الحيوانات الأهلية وأجود منها كثيرا. ثالثة الأغذية.

(٢٤) الخمر التي تمزج بمثلها ماء تسخن البدن كلّه وتتحرّك إلى جميع الأعضاء حركة
سريعة وتصلح أخلاط البدن وتجوّدها بأن تعدّل مزاجها وتستفرغ الرديء منها. في شرحه
لسابعة الفصول.

(25) Wine that is diluted and watery moistens and weakens the stomach and produces intestinal winds because of the coldness and fluidity of the water. Pure wine causes twitching[48] in the temples, heaviness in the head, and thirst because of its heat. *In Hippocratis De acutorum morborum [victu] commentarius* 2.[49]

(26) In the case of a hangover, the head is filled with vapor. Pure wine concocts these vapors and dissolves them. *In Hippocratis Epidemiarum librum* 2 *commentaria* 6.[50]

(27) We have nothing more effective and appropriate than the ingestion of wine for the case in which someone's strength has diminished, weakened, and collapsed. The same applies to someone whose entire body has become cold or whose complexion has changed. *In Hippocratis Epidemiarum librum* 6 *commentaria* 6.[51]

(28) All sweet black wines fill the vessels with thick, dark blood.[52] Thin white wines cut the thick chymes and cleanse the blood through the urine. Yellow wines are in the middle between these two and produce chymes that are intermediate in their consistency. *De victu attenuante.*[53]

(29) Thin wine is beneficial for producing good chyme and helps digestion. Yellow wine and wine that tends towards whiteness are good for stimulating micturition. *De sanitate tuenda* 4.[54]

(30)[55] Anyone whose strength needs to be revived should not drink anything but thin white wine that is pure, only contains a small amount of water, and is slightly astringent, as this is one of the most beneficial things for such a person if he does not have a fever. *De methodo [medendi]* 7.[56]

(31) Wine is one of the most appropriate things for someone who suffers from a liver affliction without an inflammation or a hot bad temperament, because it nourishes, concocts, strengthens and fights, and counteracts putrefaction. If his dyscrasia happens to be cold and moist, [wine] heals him. *Mayāmir* 8.[57]

(٢٥) الخمر الممزوجة المائية ترطّب المعدة وتضعفها وتولّد في الأمعاء رياحا لبرد الماء ورطوبته. والخمر الصرف يحدث اختلاجا في الأصداغ وثقلا في الرأس وعطشا لحرارتها. في شرحه لثانية الأمراض الحادّة.

(٢٦) الرأس في حال الخمار يمتلئ من البخار. والشراب الصرف ينضج تلك الأبخرة ويحلّلها. في سادسة شرحه لثانية أبيديميا.

(٢٧) ليس عندنا أبلغ ولا أوفق من شرب الخمر للقوة التي قد خارت وضعفت وسقطت. وكذلك لمن برد بدنه كلّه أو حال لونه. في سادسة من شرحه لسادسة أبيديميا.

(٢٨) جميع الخمور الحلوة السود تملأ العروق دما غليظا أسود. والأبيض اللطيف منها تقطع الكيموسات الغليظة وتنقّي الدم بالبول. والخمور الشقر متوسّطة تولّد كيموسا متوسّطا في قوامه. في مقالته في التدبير الملطّف.

(٢٩) الخمر الرقيقة نافعة في تولّد الكيموس المحمود معينة على الهضم والخمر الكوصية وما يضرب إلى البياض نافعتان في إدرار البول. رابعة تدبير الصحّة.

(٣٠) جميع من يحتاج إلى الإنعاش ليس ينبغي أن يشرب شيئا خلا الشراب الرقيق الأبيض الصافي القليل الاحتمال للماء الذي فيه قبض يسير. فإنّ هذا أنفع الأشياء لهم إن لم يكن ثمّ حمّى. سابعة الحيلة.

(٣١) الشراب من أوفق الأشياء لمن كانت به علّة في كبده من غير ورم أو سوء مزاج حارّ لأنّه يغذو وينضج ويقوّي ويقاوم العفونة ويضادّها. وإن اتّفق أن يكون سوء المزاج باردا رطبا شفاه. ثامنة الميامر.

---

١ وتضعفها] وتدفعها B || ٥ أبيديميا] أفيديميا ELU || ٧ أبيديميا] أفيديميا ELU || ١١ الخمور] الخمر B
تولّد] توليد L || الكوصية] القصية EL الخوصي G (= * كرصيا = κιρρός)

(32) Drinking cold water before meals is harmful for the liver, and in some people it is also harmful for the nerves.[58] *In Hippocratis De natura hominis.*[59]

(33) The worst of all waters are those derived from melted snow and ice because the fine part of rainwater dissolves but the thick, bad part freezes and never regains the excellent quality of rainwater. *De aeris [aquis locis] commentarius* 2.[60]

(34) All extremely cold water is thick and hard, slow to be digested and to pass.[61] All[62] turbid water strengthens the appetite. The reason for this is that in the summer [the turbid water] corrupts the humors so that these bite the stomach, while during winter these humors bite the cardia of the stomach because they are confined [to that place] because of the cold. *De aeris [aquis locis] commentarius* 2.

(35) Rapid transformation of water indicates its goodness and not its badness. Rainwater,[63] once it is spoiled, does not regain its [original] goodness. Therefore, one should wait until the bad smell lessens and then mix it with honey or wine; but cooking is of no use whatsoever for it. *De aeris [aquis locis] commentarius* 2.

(36) When bad water that is turbid or foul-smelling or slow to pass through the stomach or another organ is boiled, this removes its badness and makes it fit for drinking; this process should go quickly for then the water's earthern parts are separated from it and settle. Boil it at the end of the day, leave it over for the entire night, filter it, and then drink it. *In Hippocratis Epidemiarum librum* 6 *commentaria* 4.[64]

(٣٢) شرب الماء البارد قبل الطعام يضرّ بالكبد وربّما نال العصب منه مضرّة في بعض الناس. في شرحه لطبيعة الإنسان.

(٣٣) أردأ المياه كلّها التي تنحلّ من الثلج والجليد لأنّ لطيف ماء المطر قد انحلّ وجمد الغليظ الرديء ولا يعود إلى جودة ماء المطر أبدا. في شرحه لثانية المياه.

(٣٤) كلّ ماء شديد البرد فهو غليظ جاس بطيء النضج والانحدار. وكلّ ماء عكر يقوّي شهوة الغذاء وسبب ذلك في الصيف إفساده للأخلاط فتلذع المعدة وفي الشتاء لانحصار الأخلاط بالبرد تلذع فم المعدة. في شرحه لثانية من الأهوية.

(٣٥) سرعة استحالة المياه تدلّ على جودتها لا على رداءتها وماء المطر إذا عفن لا يعود إلى جودته. فلذلك ينبغي أن يصبر عليه حتّى تنفشّ عنه رائحته الرديئة ثمّ يمزج بعسل أو بشراب ولا يغني عنه الطبخ شيئا. في شرحه للثانية من الأهوية.

(٣٦) الماء الرديء الذي هو عكر أو منتن أو بطيء في المعدة أو غير ذلك إذا طبخ فإنّ الطبخ يزيل عنه رداءته ويصلحه للشرب. ويسرع انفعاله وتتميّز منه الأجزاء الأرضية وترسب فيه. فينبغي أن يطبخ آخر النهار ويترك بالليل كلّه ويصفّى ويشرب. في الرابعة من شرحه لسادسة أبيديميا.

١ بالكبد] بالمعدة والكبد L بالطعام والكبد E ‖ ٣-٤ أردأ . . . أبدا] قال بقراط أمّا المياه التي تكون من الثلوج فكلّها رديئة لأنّها إذا جمدت مرّة لم ترجع إلى طبيعتها الأولى لأنّ ما كان من الماء خفيفا عذبا صافيا نقيًّا أفلت من الجمود وطار وما كان من الماء كدرا بقي على حاله C ‖ ٥ كلّ . . . بطيء النضج] فإنّه عني به ما كان من المياه بردها شبيهة ببرد الثلوج والجليد وذلك أنّها قريبة منها وأنّها غليظة جاسية بطيئة النضج C ٥-٦ وكلّ . . . المعدة] om. C ‖ ٨ سرعة . . . رداءتها] سرعة استحالة المياه ممّا يدلّ على جودتها لا على رداءتها C ‖ ٨-١٠ وماء . . . شيئا] إنّ هذا الماء إذا بدأ يعفن ويفسد فإنّه لم يغن عنه الطبخ شيئا فينبغي أن يصير له شيء ينفّس العفونة عنه . . . فيخلط لذلك معه عسل مطبوخ منزوع الرغوة C ‖ ١٤ أبيديميا] أفيديميا ELU

(37) Rainwater does not change into another kind of putrefying quality.[65] If you do not have rainwater available, be satisfied with spring water, for it is sufficient when this water is clean and pure. *Mayāmir* 7.[66]

(38) The best water is that in which no taste nor odor is perceptible. This water is the sweetest and most delicious [to drink]. Any water that streams towards the east over clean sand and that quickly warms and cools is the best water for[67] anyone [whatever his age]. *De sanitate tuenda* 1.[68]

(39) Milk nourishes an emaciated body and revives it. It hinders the bad humors from causing harm and even improves them. It softens the stools. But cheese settles in the passages of the liver and obstructs them and is therefore very harmful for dropsy patients. *In Hippocratis Epidemiarum librum* 2 *commentaria* 6.[69]

(40) In book 4 of [his commentary on Hippocrates'] *De alimento*, he says that milk is more nutritious than wheat[70] [*Triticum vulgare* and var.]. And in *De bonis [malisque] sucis*, he says that milk is the best thing in producing good chymes.[71]

(41) Watery moisture prevails in the milk of camels and donkeys, cheesy moisture prevails in sheep's milk, and fat in cow's milk. Compared to the milk of other animals, goat's milk is intermediate between these unbalanced conditions. It is also intermediate in its effect on the human body. The milk that produces the best chyme (if one drinks it immediately after milking) comes from an animal that is healthy and in a good condition. One acts prudently if one adds a small amount of honey and salt to be sure that it does not turn into cheese. *De bonis [malisque] sucis.*[72]

(42) As for milk that seems to have curdled[73]—and the most curdled kind of milk is cheese—it is one of the things that is extremely thickening when it is eaten dry. Milk that is greatly dominated by the cheesy part, such as cow's milk and sheep's milk, is the thickest of all [kinds of

(٣٧) ماء القطر لا يتغيّر إلى كيفية أخرى من جنس العفونة. ومتى لم تقدر على ماء القطر فاقتصر على ماء العيون لأنّه يكتفي من الماء بأن يكون نقيا صافيا. سابعة الميامر.

(٣٨) أفضل المياه ما لا يتبيّن له طعم ولا رائحة وهذا الماء أعذب ماء وألذّ. وكلّ ماء يجري نحو المشرق على تربة نقية ويسخن سريعا ويبرد سريعا فهو أصلح المياه لجميع الإنسان. الأولى من تدبير الصحّة. ٥

(٣٩) اللبن يغذو البدن المنهوك وينعشه ويكسر من عادية الأخلاط الرديئة حتّى يعدّلها ويلين البطن. والجبن يرسخ في مجاري الكبد ويسدّها ولذلك هو من أضرّ شيء لأصحاب الاستسقاء. في سادسة شرحه لثانية أبيديميا.

(٤٠) وقال في الرابعة من كتاب الغذاء إنّ اللبن أكثر غذاء من القمح. وقال في مقالته في جودة الكيموس إنّ اللبن أحسن الأشياء كلّها كيموسا. ١٠

(٤١) الأغلب على لبن اللقاح والأتن الرطوبة المائية وعلى لبن النعاج الجبنية وعلى لبن البقر الدسم. وأمّا لبن الماعز فهو وسط بين الحالات المجاوزة للاعتدال إذا قيس بسائر ألبان الحيوان وهو متوسّط في فعله في بدن الإنسان وأفضله في جودة الكيموس ما كان من الحيوان الخصب الصحيح البدن إذا شرب ساعة يحلب. ومن الحزم أن يلقى فيه عسل وملح يسير ليأمن من التجبّن. في مقالته في جودة الكيموس. ١٥

(٤٢) وأمّا اللبن فكأنّه مغلّظ وأكثر من اللبن تغليظا الجبن وهو من الأشياء التي تغلّظ غاية التغليظ متى أكل يابسا. وما غلب عليه من الألبان الجزء الجبني غلبة شديدة مثل لبن

١ القطر] المطر EL || ٢ القطر] المطر EL | نّه] فإنّه BELU || ٣ لا] لم BL || ٤ الإنسان] الناس L ||
٨ أبيديميا] أفيديميا ELU || ١١ الأغلب] يغلب EL | والأتن] والأتان EL || ١٥ من التجبّن] ألا يتجبّن L
التجبّن EU || ١٦ تغليظا] غلظا L

milk]. The thinnest [milk] is that in which the watery part dominates, such as the milk of donkeys, for if it is taken with honey or salt, it does not harm someone who needs a thinning diet. But one should be on one's guard against the other kinds of milk. *De bonis [malisque] sucis.*[74]

(43) Cow's milk is the thickest and fattest of all sorts of milk, while that of camels is the moistest of all sorts of milk with the least amount of fat. After camel's milk is mare's milk, and after that is donkey's milk. Goat's milk is intermediate between thick and thin milk, but sheep's milk is thicker than it. *De alimentorum [facultatibus]* 3.[75]

(44) All sorts of milk are good and beneficial for[76] the chest and lungs, but they are not suitable for the head unless the head is extremely strong. Milk is unsuitable for[77] the [parts below the cartilage of the] ribs since these are easily filled with flatulence. *De alimentorum [facultatibus]* 3.[78]

(45) The best sort of cheese is the fresh one that is made from milk from which the fat has been removed. This cheese is the most delicious of all sorts of cheeses and does not harm the stomach. It is the most rapid sort of cheese to pass and[79] does not provide bad nutrition nor unwholesome blood [as all other cheeses do]. *De alimentorum [facultatibus]* 3.[80]

(46) The foods that are extremely weak are vegetables and most fruits that are surrounded by a hard shell. These have the property to weaken the body, and if one uses them constantly, one shortens one's life. *In Hippocratis Epidemiarum librum 6 commentaria* 5.[81]

(47) Vegetables do not have good chymes. Lettuce[82] [*Lactuca sativa*] is a cooling vegetable that is harmless; turnip[83] [*Brassica rapa*] is between good and bad, and after it Jew's mallow [*Corchorus olitorius*], and then orache [*Atriplex hortensis*], purslane [*Portulaca oleracea*], and purple amaranth [*Amaranthus blitum*]. *De bonis [malisque] sucis.*[84]

البقر ولبن النعاج فهو أغلظها كلّها. وألطفها ما غلب عليه الجزء المائي مثل لبن الأتن فإنّه إن

اتّخذ بعسل أو ملح فليس يضرّ من كان يحتاج إلى التدبير اللطيف. وأمّا سائر الألبان فينبغي

أن يتحفّظ منها. في تلك المقالة.

(٤٣) لبن البقر أغلظ الألبان كلّها وأدسمها ولبن الإبل أرطب الألبان كلّها وأقلّها دسما.

وبعد لبن الإبل الخيل وبعده لبن الأتن ولبن الماعز معتدل بين الغليظ والرقيق ولبن النعاج ٥

أغلظ منه. ثالثة الأغذية.

(٤٤) الألبان كلّها جيّدة صالحة لمواضع الصدر والرئة وغير موافقة للرأس إلّا أن يكون

قويا جدًّا. ولا اللبن موافق للجنبين إذا كانت النفخة تسرع إليهمًا. ثالثة الأغذية.

(٤٥) أفضل أصناف الجبن الحديث الذي عمل من اللبن الذي أزيل زبده وهذا الجبن ألذّ

أصناف الجبن كلّها وغير ضارّ للمعدة وأسرع أصنافه انحدارا وليس برديء الغذاء ولا يولّد ١٠

دما غير محمود. ثالثة الأغذية.

(٤٦) الأطعمة التي هي في غاية الضعف هي البقول وأكثر الثمار التي يحويها قشر

صلب. ومن شأن هذه أن تضعف البدن وإن أدمن عليها قصّرت العمر. في الخامسة من

شرحه لسادسة أبيديميا.

(٤٧) البقول ليس فيها حسن الكيموس والخسّ بقلة مبرّدة غير ضارّة واللفت فيما بين ١٥

الجيّد والرديء وبعده الملوخيا وبعده القطف والبقلة الحمقاء والبقلة اليمانية. في مقالته في

جودة الكيموس.

٩ ألذّ] أجود L || ١٠ للمعدة] بالمعدة BELU || ١٤ أبيديميا] أفيديميا ELU || ١٦ الملوخيا] الملوكيا L

الملوكية O | في مقالته في جودة الكيموس] في تلك المقالة G

(48) If cucumber and watermelon are not quickly passed, they corrupt in the stomach and the chyme resulting from [the putrefaction] is almost a fatal poison. *De bonis [malisque] sucis.*[85]

(49) Thinning vegetables[86] are garlic [*Allium sativum*], onion [*Alllium cepa*], garden cress [*Lepidium sativum* L.], leek [*Allium porrum* and var.], and mustard [*Brassica alba* var. *nigra*]. [Next in strength] after these come parsley[87] [*Petroselinum* spp.], fennel [*Foeniculum vulgare*], mountain mint[88] [perhaps *Nepeta cataria* and var.], water mint [*Mentha aquatica*], oregano,[89] lesser calamint [*Clinopodium nepeta* and var.],[90] bishop's weed [*Ammi visnaga*], and Massilian hartwort [*Seseli tortuosum* L.], when these are taken fresh.[91] [Next in strength] after these come rocket [*Eruca sativa*], water parsnip[92] (that is, water celery [perhaps *Sium latifolium* or *Apium inundatum* or *Apium nodiflorum* and var.]), garden celery, the seed[93] of mountain celery [*Peucedanum oreoselinum* Moensch], basil [*Ocimum basilicum*], radish, cabbage [*Brassica oleracea*], blackberry[94] [Br. bramble; *Rubus fruticosus*], and other types of fragrant and sharp plants. *De victu attenuante.*[95]

(50) Poppy [*Papaver somniferum* and var.] seeds are much less cooling than the plants, so one can sprinkle them on bread and mix them with many other foods that one prepares without causing any harm. But they do cause heaviness in the head and induce sleep. Sesame [*Sesamum indicum*] [seeds] produce thick and sticky chymes in the body. *De victu attenuante.*[96]

(51) All fruits from trees, with a few exceptions, produce bad chymes. Such an exception is the [fruit from the] chestnut tree [*Castanea sativa*], because in spite of its thickness, it does not produce any bad chyme if it is well digested. All fresh fruits produce bad chymes, and if they spoil in the stomach, they cause fatal poisoning. Figs and grapes are less bad. Dried figs together with walnuts [*Juglans regia*] and almonds [*Prunus amygdalis*] have beneficial chymes. *De bonis [malisque] sucis.*[97]

(52) Fresh, ripe figs are among the intermediate foods about which one can say neither that they have a thinning effect on the chymes nor that they have a thickening effect on them.[98] Those apples [*Malus sylvestris* and var.] and pears [*Pyrus communis*] that are eaten when they are cooked are less harmful than those that are eaten while they are raw.[99] *De victu attenuante.*

(٤٨) القِثّاء والبطّيخ إن لم ينحدر سريعا فإنّه يفسد في البطن فيصير الكيموس المتولّد منه قريبا من السموم القتّالة. في مقالته في جودة الكيموس.

(٤٩) الأشياء الملطّفة الثوم والبصل والحرف والكرّاث والخردل وبعد هذه المقدونس والرازيانج والفوذنج الجبلي والنهري والصعتر والحاشا والنانخواه والساليوس إذا أكلت وهي طرية. وبعده الجرجير وقرّة العين وهو كرفس الماء والكرفس البستاني والفطراساليون والباذروج والفجل والكرنب والعلّيق وسائر أصناف النبات الطيّبة الرائحة الحرّيفة. في مقالته في التدبير الملطّف.

(٥٠) بزر الخشخاش أقلّ بردا من نبات الخشخاش بكثير حتّى أنّه ينثر على الخبز ويخلط بكثير ممّا يحضر حتّى كأنّه لا مضرّة فيه ويحدث في الرأس ثقلا وينوّم. والسمسم يولّد في البدن كيموسا غليظا لزجا. في تلك المقالة.

(٥١) ثمر الشجر كلّه إلّا القليل منه رديء الكيموس إلّا الشاهبلّوط فإنّه مع غلظه إن انهضم جيّدا لم يكن له كيموس رديء. والفاكهة الرطبة كلّها رديئة الكيموس و إن فسدت في المعدة أورثت السموم القتّالة. والتين والعنب أقلّها رداءة. والتين اليابس مع الجوز واللوز محمود الكيموس. في مقالته في جودة الكيموس.

(٥٢) التين الرطب ما كان منه نضجا فهو من الأغذية المتوسّطة التي لا يمكن أن يقال فيها إنّها تلطّف الكيموسات ولا تغلّظها. وما أكل من التفّاح أو الكمّثراء وقد طبخ أقلّ ضررا ممّا يؤكل منها وهي نيئة. في مقالته في التدبير الملطّف.

---

٢ في مقالته في جودة الكيموس] في تلك المقالة EL ‖ ٤ والصعتر] والزعتر U ‖ والساليوس] والسفاليوس LO وسائر أصناف النبات الطيّبة الرائحة الحرّيفة] .add GU¹ ‖ ٥ وبعده] وبعد هذه BELU ‖ والفطراساليون] والبطرساليون EL ‖ ٦ وسائر ... الحرّيفة] G¹ ‖ ١٢ له كيموس رديء] كيموسا رديئا BELU ‖ ١٤ في مقالته في جودة الكيموس] في تلك المقالة L

(53) If[100] mulberries [*Morus alba* var. *nigra*] do not pass quickly, they spoil in the stomach in an extraordinary, unusual way that is beyond description, just like watermelons and gourds[101] when they are not passed. For although gourds are the most harmless of the summer fruits, when they are not passed from the stomach quickly, they cause severe corruption. *De alimentorum [facultatibus]* 2.[102]

(54) All dates are hard to digest and cause headache and [a sensation of] sharpness[103] and biting at the cardia of the stomach when one eats too many of them. Unripe dates fill the body with crude, raw humors that obstruct the liver and cause shivering and rigor that is difficult to warm. *De alimentorum [facultatibus]* 2.[104]

(55) He says in *Mayāmir*, book 2: "Palm dates have a specific[105] property that causes headache."[106]

(56) Olives strengthen the stomach and whet the appetite. The olives most suited to this task are those that are preserved in vinegar. Walnuts are more rapidly digested than hazelnuts [*Corylus avellana*] but are less nutritious. They are better for the stomach than hazelnuts, especially when they are eaten together with dried figs. *De alimentorum [facultatibus]* 2.[107]

(57) Raisins are hardly susceptible to putrefaction. In general, their[108] substance is similar and conformable to the nature of the liver. They cure its bad temperament, nourish it, concoct the unconcocted humors, and correct[109] the bad humors and improve their temperament. For this reason they are extremely valuable for healing these sorts of illnesses. *Mayāmir* 8.[110]

(58) The foods that are most[111] similar to blood are those that are intermediate between thin and thick. These include the good types of bread; the meat of chickens, partridges, pigeons, turtledoves, francolins, [and] pheasants; all sorts of fish that do not contain stickiness or grease or [have a] repulsive taste; and[112] gently boiled eggs. *De bonis [malisque] sucis*.[113]

The best food that does not have any clear medicinal power nor a very nutritious substance is barley gruel that has been well prepared, and after it barley groats. After these comes gruel[114] from wheat or spelt

(٥٣) التوت إذا لم ينحدر سريعا فسد في المعدة فسادا غربيا نادرا لا ينطق به على مثال فساد البطّيخ والقرع إذا لم ينحدر فإنّ القرع مع كونه أقلّ الثمار الصيفية مضرّة متى لم ينحدر عن المعدة سريعا فسد فسادا عظيما. ثانية الأغذية.

(٥٤) جميع التمر عسر الانهضام يحدث صداعا عند الإكثار من أكله ويبثر فم المعدة ويلذعه. والبسر يملأ البدن خلطا نيئا خاما ويحدث قشعريرة ونافضا عسر ما يسخن ويسدّد الكبد. ثانية الأغذية.

(٥٥) وقال في الثانية للميامر: تمر النخل فيه خاصّية يؤلم بها الرأس ويصدعه.

(٥٦) الزيتون يقوّي المعدة ويفتق الشهوة وأجوده لذلك المخلّل. والجوز أسرع انهضاما من البندق وأقلّ غذاء وأوفق من البندق للمعدة وخاصّة إذا أكل مع التين اليابس. ثانية الأغذية.

(٥٧) الزبيب عسر ما يقبل العفونة وجملة جوهره مشاكل للكبد مخصوصا بها يشفي سوء مزاجها ويغذوها وينضج الأخلاط التي لم تنضج ويعدّل الأخلاط الرديئة ويصلح مزاجها. وهذا جليل القدر في علاج أمثال هذه العلل. ثامنة الميامر.

(٥٨) أقرب الأطعمة من الدم هي المتوسّطة بين اللطيفة والغليظة وهي أنواع الخبز المحمود ولحمان الدجاج والحجل والحمام واليمام والدرّاج والتدرج وجميع السمك الذي ليس فيه لزوجة ولا زفورة ولا بشاعة والبيض الرعّاد. في مقالته في جودة الكيموس.

الأغذية التي ليس فيها شيء ظاهر من قوى الأدوية ولا فيها من الجوهر الغاذي مقدار كثير جدّا أفضلها ماء كشك الشعير المحكم الصنعة وبعده كشك الشعير وبعده الخندروس

١ ينطق به] ينطبق B ‖ ٥ والبسر] والبصل L ‖ ويسدّد] ويسدّ L ‖ ٧ للميامر] الميامر BELOU ‖ النخل] النخيل L ‖ ٩ من البندق] منه L ‖ ١٣ علاج] om. ELOU ‖ ثامنة] ثانية BGL

with a small amount of vinegar, and gruel from wheat or spelt with no vinegar [at all]. Bread baked in an oven[115] is also good foodstuff, and of the fishes all those[116] that live among the rocks. The best [kinds of] birds are the partridge[117] and mountain sparrows. After these come chickens and francolins. Those animals that are very old or young (that is, just born) should be avoided. *De methodo [medendi]* 8.[118]

(59) Foods that produce thick, sticky chyme are very nutritious. If they are well digested in the stomach and liver, they produce beneficial blood. Only someone who performs strenuous physical exercise before his meals should take these foods. But someone who merely looks after the health of his body and not after its vigor[119] should guard against all foods that produce thick chyme and should avoid thickening foods even if they have beneficial chymes. *De bonis [malisque] sucis.*[120]

(60) Thick, sticky foods include [all][121] types of bread whose baking was bad—that is, bread that was not well leavened or was insufficiently salted, kneaded, or baked—also[122] all types of cheese, roasted or hard-boiled eggs, [all] types of large fish with hard, sticky meat, mushrooms and truffles, large pine nuts, and palm dates. Lentils, cabbage, acorns [*Quercus* and var.], and chestnuts are not sticky, although they produce thick chymes. *De bonis [malisque] sucis.*[123]

(61) All people should always avoid foods with bad chymes, except for those who work hard during the summer and need to treat the dry-ness and heat of their bodies. In such a situation it is appropriate for them to eat mulberries, plums, cherries, cucumbers, watermelons, apri-cots, or peaches before their meal, and also cooled milk and gourds. If a person practices[124] moderation in his lifestyle, he can cool and moisten [the dryness and heat] resulting from his hard work with another kind of regimen, namely by going to the bathhouse and by feeding himself thereafter with foods that have good chymes and that are seasoned with vinegar and the like. *De bonis [malisque] sucis.*[125]

بخلّ يسير وبعده الخندروس بلا خلّ، وخبز التنّور أيضا طعام جيّد. ومن السمك جميع ما هو رضراضي. وأفضل الطيور الطيهوج والعصافير الجبلية وبعدها الدجاج والدرّاج. ويجتنب من الحيوان الهرم وطرئة القريب بالولادة. ثامنة الحيلة.

(٥٩) الأطعمة التي تولّد كيموسا غليظا لزجا فهي كثيرة الغذاء جدّا. وإن هي انهضمت في المعدة والكبد انهضاما جيّدا ولّدت دما محمودا ولا ينبغي أن يستعملها إلّا من يرتاض قبل طعامه رياضة قوية. ومن كان يعني بأمر صحّة بدنه لا بخصبه ويحذر من الأطعمة كلّما يولّد كيموسا غليظا ويجتنب الأغذية الغليظة ولو كانت محمودة الكيموس. في مقالته في جودة الكيموس.

(٦٠) الأطعمة الغليظة اللزجة أنواع الخبز الرديء الصنعة أعني ما لم يختمر حسنا أو الناقص الملح أو الناقص النضج أو الناقص الدعك والأجبان كلّها والبيض الذي قد شوي أو طبخ حتّى صلب وأنواع الأسماك الكبيرة الجرم والصلبة اللحم واللزجة والفطر والكمأة وحبّ الصنوبر الكبار وتمر النخل. وأمّا العدس والكرنب والبلّوط والقسطل فإنّها غير لزجة وإن كانت غليظة الكيموس. في مقالته في جودة الكيموس.

(٦١) الأغذية الرديئة الكيموس ينبغي للناس كلّهم أن يجتنبوها أبدا إلّا أن تعبوا في الصيف فيحتاجون إلى مداواة يبس أبدانهم وحرارتها فيصلح لهم عند ذلك أن يأكلوا قبل الطعام التوت أو الإجّاص أو القراصيا أو القثّاء أو البطّيخ أو المشمش أو الخوخ واللبن المبرّد أيضا والقرع. وإذا كان الرجل عفيفا في تدبيره مجتهدا فقد يمكنه أن يبرد ويرطّب ما حدث من التعب بضرب آخر من التدبير بدخول الحمّام ويغتذي بعده بأغذية جيّدة الكيموس مطيّبة بخلّ ونحو ذلك. في مقالته في جودة الكيموس.

(62) Food that is hard to dissolve is that consisting of thick, sticky things such as pork and pure[126] bread. If someone who does not exercise were to constantly eat this food, he would soon suffer from the illness of overfilling, just as if someone who practices bodily exercise were to constantly feed himself with vegetables and barley juice, his body would be destroyed and quickly waste away. *De alimentorum [facultatibus]* 1.[127]

(63) Everything that is moister in its consistency provides the body with little nourishment. It dissolves and evaporates rapidly and is easily digested so that the body needs other, new food. But everything that is hard and earth-like provides the body with rich, lasting nourishment that is difficult to dissolve and evaporate and is not easily digested nor converted into blood. *De alimentorum [facultatibus]* 1.[128]

(64) One should bear in mind a factor common to all foods: whatever is sharp and spicy or bitter provides little nourishment, while whatever is tasteless provides the body with rich nourishment; even more so whatever is sweet, especially when its substance is solid. [This[129] is the case] whether these flavors are natural or acquired through preparation—that is, through cooking, roasting, frying, macerating in water, and the like. *De alimentorum [facultatibus]* 2.[130]

(65) Things that are greasy and sticky, such[131] as the [different kinds of] fat, satiate and fill someone who eats them from the outset, as soon as they reach the stomach. And then they diminish and lessen his appetite. A human being cannot bear to eat such food constantly. *De alimentorum [facultatibus]* 3.[132]

(66) Something that is truly sweet is undoubtedly nutritious. But something bitter is not nutritious, and something with an intermediate flavor is less nutritious than something sweet. The same holds true for the other flavors because they are not nutritious, with the only exception of the sweet flavor. And also something fatty is of the [same] kind as something sweet and is nutritious. *De [simplicium] medicamentorum [temperamentis ac facultatibus]* 4.[133]

(٦٢) الغذاء العسر التحلّل هو غذاء الأشياء الغليظة اللزجة مثل غذاء لحم الخنزير والخبز النقي ولو أنّ من لا يقرب الرياضة دام على استعمال هذا الغذاء لأسرع إليه مرض الامتلاء كما أنّ من يعالج الرياضة لو دام على الاغتذاء بالبقول وماء الشعير لفسد بدنه وأسرع إليه السلّ. أوّل الأغذية.

(٦٣) كلّما كان الشيء أرطب قواما كان ما يناله البدن منه من الغذاء يسيرا سريع التحلّل والتهبي ويسهل انهضامه فيحتاج البدن إلى غذاء آخر مجدّد. وكلّما كان صلبا أرضيا فيغذو البدن غذاء كثيرا لابثا عسر التحلّل والتهبّي وليس يسهل الانهضام والاستحالة إلى الدم. أوّل الأغذية. ٥

(٦٤) ينبغي أن تذكر في جميع الأطعمة عامّة أنّ ما كان منها حرّيفا حادّا أو مرّا فغذاؤه يسير. وما كان منها لا طعم له فما يصل من غذائه إلى البدن كثير وأكثر منه ما كان حلوا ولا سيّما إن كان جرمه ملزّزا سوى كانت هذه الطعوم بالطبع أو مكتسبة بالصنعة أعني الطبخ والشيّ والقلي والنقيع في الماء ونحو ذلك. ثانية الأغذية. ١٠

(٦٥) الأشياء التي لها دسم ولزوجة كالشحوم ساعة تصل إلى المعدة في أوّل ما تؤكل تشبع وتملأ جوف الآكل لها. ثمّ ترجع وتقلّل شهوته وتقصّرها. والإنسان لا يصبر على مداومتها. ثالثة الأغذية. ١٥

(٦٦) الشيء الصادق الحلاوة يغذو لا محالة والشيء المرّ لا يغذو والشيء الذي هو في ما بينهما في الطعم غذاؤه أقلّ من غذاء الشيء الحلو. وكذلك الحال في سائر الطعوم الأُخَر لأنّها لا تغذو خلا الطعم الحلو فقط والشيء الدسم أيضا هو من جنس العذب الحلو ويغذو. رابعة *الأدوية.

٣ لو] om. L ‖ ٥ منه] om. LU ‖ ١٧ في الطعم] بالطبع BELOU غذاؤه] G¹ ‖ لأنّها] G¹ ‖
١٩ *الأدوية] الأغذية MSS

(67) Says Moses: Abū Marwān b. Zuhr[134] mentions the benefits of some foods that[135] have been confirmed by testing. These foods work through specific properties. He mentions them in the *Book*[136] *on Foods*, which he composed for one of the Almoravid kings. Some of these were mentioned by his father in his *Tadhkira*.[137] It seems me to me a good thing to write them down in [the form of] aphorisms, and they are the following:

(68)[138] Boiled chicken soup balances the temperament. It is the best medicine and foodstuff for the beginning of elephantiasis. It[139] fattens the body of the emaciated and convalescents. Young doves have the special property of producing migraine, especially their necks. Turtledoves increase memory, sharpen the intellect, and strengthen the senses. Partridges, when boiled, cause constipation, but if they are boiled in their skins, they relieve the bowels. Similarly, hens[140] and[141] roosters are very effective in relieving the bowels.

(69)[142] Sparrows[143] are beneficial for paralysis,[144] hemiplegia, facial paresis, and the different kinds of dropsy, and [also] increase sexual potency. Domesticated pigeons that live together and[145] fly around freely increase the innate heat. Soup [made] from larks loosens a colic. The nature of quails is close to that of sparrows; its [meat] is beneficial for healthy people and convalescents; its substance is fine; it dissolves kidney stones and stimulates micturition.

(70)[146] He says: The meat of kids is different from that of all other quadrupeds because it is exceedingly good. The meat of gazelles[147] has the special property of strengthening the soul, and the juice of its meat revives someone whose strength has collapsed and resuscitates[148] someone who has fainted because of excessive evacuation.

(71)[149] The testicles of roosters provide extremely good nourishment and are the best food one can give to emaciated people and convalescents. All testicles of living creatures are hot and moist and clearly help sexual potency.

(72)[150] Pigeon eggs improve sexual potency and are beneficial to it. All eggs improve sexual potency, especially when they are boiled with onion or turnip.[151]

(٦٧) قال موسى: ذكر أبو مروان بن زهر منافع قد صحّت تجربتها في بعض الأغذية وتجري مجرى الخواصّ وذكرها في كتابه الذي ألّفه في الأغذية لأحد ملوك المرابطين وذكر بعضها أبوه في تذكرة له. وقد حسن عندي تقييدها في فصول وهي هذه:

(٦٨) أمراق الدجاج المسلوقة تعدّل المزاج وهي أفضل دواء وغذاء في ابتداء الجذام وتخصّب جسم المنهوكين والناقهين. وفراخ الحمام لها خاصّية في توليد الشقيقة ولا سيّما أعناقها. واليمام يزيد في الحفظ ويذكي الذهن ويقوّي الحواسّ. والحجل مسلوقة تمسك الطبع و إذا سلقت بجلودها أطلقت الطبع. وكذلك الدجاج والديوك أبلغ في إطلاق البطن.

(٦٩) العصافير نافعة من الاسترخاء والفالج واللقوة وأنواع الاستسقاء وتزيد في قوة الجماع. الحمام الأهلية الراعية الناهضة تنمي الحرارة الغريزية. أمراق القنابر تطلق القولنج. والسمّان قريبة من طبيعة العصافير نافعة للأصحّاء والناقهين لطيفة الجوهر تفتّت الحصى وتدرّ البول.

(٧٠) قال: لحوم الجداء كادت تخرج لإفراطها في الجودة عن لحوم ذوات الأربع. لحم الغزال له خاصّية في تقوية النفس وماء لحمه ينعش من سقطت قوته ويبرئ من غشي عليه من كثرة الاستفراغ.

(٧١) أخصية الديوك محمودة الغذاء جدّا وهي أفضل ما يغذى به المنهوكون والناقهون. وجميع أخصية الحيوان حارّة رطبة وتعين على الباه معونة ظاهرة.

(٧٢) بيض الحمام يعين على الجماع معونة صالحة وجميع البيض يعين على الجماع وبخاصّة إذا طبخت بالبصل واللفت.

١ صحّت تجربتها] جرّبها BEL جرّبها OU || ٤ في ابتداء] لابتداء BELOU || ٩ الناهضة] التي تأوي في الأبراج Ibn Zuhr | القنابر] القنبر L || ١٣ له] G¹ | ويبرئ] G¹ || ١٧ معونة صالحة وجميع البيض يعين على الجماع] G¹

(73)¹⁵² In general, all [types of] milk relieve the bowels, and camel milk strengthens the stomach and liver. Raisins fatten the liver and are beneficial for it through their special property. Unripe, sour grapes strengthen the stomach through their special property and by virtue of their nature balance the temperament of those suffering from heat. They stop [the urge to] vomit in an amazing way when it is caused by yellow bile.

(74)¹⁵³ The smell of an apple strengthens the heart and the brain and is beneficial for those suffering from marasmus and delusions. However, as to its [actual] consumption, he states that it is more harmful than the consumption of any other fruit because its fragrance gives rise to gases in the nerves and¹⁵⁴ in the muscles that can only be dissolved with difficulty.

(75)¹⁵⁵ Pears strengthen the stomach and have the special property of quenching thirst when eaten after a meal. If one lets their juice stand, it turns into a vinegar that strengthens the stomach in a wonderful way and does not harm the nerves because of the astringency and fragrance that it contains.

(76)¹⁵⁶ When eaten with bread, sweet pomegranates have a wonderful and special property that prevents the bread from spoiling in the stomach. Similarly, if¹⁵⁷ sour pomegranates [*Punica granatum* L. and var.] are cooked with food, that food does not spoil in the stomach.

(77)¹⁵⁸ Excessive consumption of walnuts causes stuttering; therefore, children should not eat them. Almonds induce regular sleep. If¹⁵⁹ used for cooking, they provide primarily moisture [without any superfluities]. Their oil, if trickled into the nose, induces sleep and is good for cooking.

(78)¹⁶⁰ Pistachio nuts [*Pistacia vera*] are the most salutary of fruits; they strengthen the stomach and the liver by their special property. Their oil has the same effect if rubbed on the stomach and liver. They are beneficial in many ways. If they are eaten either alone or with raisins and sugar before the meal, during the meal, or after the meal, they are beneficial for all conditions. They are of moderate heat and dryness.

(۷۳) الألبان كلّها عموما تطلق البطن ولبن النوق يقوّي المعدة والكبد. والزبيب يخصّب الكبد وينفعها بخاصّية فيه والحصرم يقوّي المعدة بخاصّية فيه ويعدّل مزاج المحرورين بطبيعته ويقطع القيء قطعا عجيبا إذا كان من صفراء.

(۷٤) التفّاح شمّه يقوّي القلب والدماغ وينفع شمّه المذبولين والموسوسين. وأمّا أكله قال فإنّه أضرّ من كلّ ما يؤكل من الفاكهة لأنّه بعطريته تتولّد منه رياح في العصب والعضل بكدّ ما تتحلّل.

(۷٥) الكمّثراء يقوّي المعدة وله خاصّية في قطع العطش إذا أكل بعد الطعام وعصيره إذا ترك خلّا صار يقوّي المعدة تقوية عجيبة ولا يضرّ بالعصب من أجل ما فيه من القبض والعطرية.

(۷٦) الرمّان الحلو له خاصّية عجيبة إذا أكل بالخبز فإنّه يمنعه من الفساد في المعدة. وكذلك الحامض إذا طبخ بالطعام لا يفسد ذلك الطعام في المعدة.

(۷۷) الإكثار من أكل الجوز يوجب التوقّف في الكلام، فلذلك ينبغي أن لا يتناول منه الصبيان. أكل اللوز ينوّم تنويما معتدلا والطبخ به يرطّب رطوبة أصلية ودهنه إذا قطّر في الأنف نوّم والطبخ به محمود.

(۷۸) الفستق أفضل الفواكه يقوّي المعدة والكبد بخاصّية فيه وكذلك دهنه يدهن به المعدة والكبد ومنافعه كثيرة وإن أكل وحده أو مع زبيب وسكّر قبل الطعام أو معه أو بعده جيّد في جميع الحالات وحرّه ويبسه معتدل.

---

٤ والموسوسين] والمنهوكين ELO المنفوسين U || ٥ والعضل] وأوجاعا في العضل Ibn Zuhr || ۱۱ إذا طبخ بالطعام لا يفسد ذلك الطعام في المعدة] فإن اتخذ رب كان نافعا من فساد الأطعمة في المعدة Ibn Zuhr || ۱۳ والطبخ به يرطّب رطوبة أصلية] إذا وضع في الطعام أحدث فيه رطوبة غير فضلية Ibn Zuhr || ۱٥ الفستق] اللوز ELO || ۱٦ وإن أكل] أكل ELOU يؤكل B

(79)[161] Dates obstruct the liver and cause an inflammation in the head. They have bad chymes; the fresh ones are much more detrimental than the dried ones and[162] have the special property of producing hemorrhoids. The hearts of the date palm (that is, its pith) produce much sperm and help sexual potency.

(80)[163] Sesame injures the brain and the spinal cord and fills the head with superfluities. It makes the mouth stink, putrefies the sweat, makes women sterile, fattens[164] the abdomen, and sometimes causes a scrotal hernia.

(81)[165] Raw or cooked cabbage purifies the voice and removes hoarseness. Eggplant [*Solanum melongena*], as a drug, strengthens, fortifies, and reinforces the stomach and is good against nausea and vomiting. But [cabbage and eggplant] are the worst of all foods and produce a large quantity of black bile. This is the end of the text [quoted] from Ibn Zuhr.

(82) Says Moses: This man who was on the Temple Mount and whose name is al-Tamīmī and who composed a book on drugs and called it *Al-murshid* [The guide], allegedly had much experience.[166] Although most of his statements are taken from others and although sometimes he wrongly understands the words of others, he still, in general, mentions many properties of various foods and medications, and therefore I decided to write down those that are good in my opinion, whether foods or medications.[167]

(83) From his statement about the special properties of foods: Eating a handful of sweetened, salted lupini [beans] [*Lupinus albus*] every day together with the skins strengthens one's vision by virtue of their special property. He further states: Young chickens that[168] are separated from their mother alleviate the heat that occurs in the cardia of the stomach. Soup[169] prepared from old roosters is good for chronic phlegmatic fevers and for asthma. Oregano has a special property of strengthening vision and is good for [weak vision] arising from moisture. It is also beneficial for scorpion stings.

(84) Orache has a special property of being good for jaundice caused by obstruction of the liver. Spinach [*Spinacia oleracea*] is beneficial for pleurisy and for any tumor that arises from yellow bile or blood. Purple amaranth[170] has the special property of eliminating thirst caused by

(٧٩) التمر يسدّد الكبد ويورم الرأس رديء الكيموس ورطبه شرّ من يابسه بكثير وله
خصوصية بتوليد البواسير. وقلب النخلة وهو الجمّار يولّد منيا كثيرا ويعين على الجماع.

(٨٠) السمسم يخلّ بالدماغ والنخاع ويملأ الرأس فضولا ويبخّر الفم وينتن العرق ويعقّم
النساء ويعظم الجوف وربّما أحدث الأدرة.

(٨١) الكرنب نيئا كان أو مطبوخا يصفّي الصوت ويزيل بحح الصياح. الباذنجان يدبغ ٥
المعدة ويشدّها ويقوّيها وينفع من التهوّع والقيء على جهة الدواء وهما أردأ الأغذية وأشرّها
وهما يولّدان السوداء توليدا عظيما. هنا انتهى كلام بن زهر.

(٨٢) قال موسى: هذا الرجل الذي كان في جبال القدس المعروف بالتميمي الذي ألّف
في الأدوية كتابا وسمّاه المرشد هو يقال كان كثير التجربة وإن كان أكثر ما يقول حكاية
عن غيره وربّما يخطئ فيما يفهم من كلام الغير لكنّه بالجملة ذكر خواصّا كثيرة لأغذية ما ١٠
ولأدوية رأيت تقييد ما حسن عندي منها في الأغذية والأدوية.

(٨٣) من كلامه في خواصّ الأغذية قال: الترمس المحلّى المملّح إذا أكل كلّ يوم منه بقشره
ملء كفّ قوّى النور الباصر بخاصّية فيه. وقال: الفراريج المحتلمة تسكن الحرارة العارضة
في فم المعدة. ومرق الديك العتيق ينفع الحمّيات البلغمية المتقادمة وينفع من الربو. الصعتر له
خاصّية في تقوية النور الباصر وينفع من ضعفه الكائن عن رطوبة وينفع من لسع العقرب. ١٥

(٨٤) القطف له خاصّية في النفع من اليرقان الكائن عن سدد الكبد. والاسفاناخ
ينفع ذات الجنب وكلّ ورم حادث عن صفراء أو دم. واليربوز له خاصّية في قطع العطش

١ وله خصوصية بتوليد البواسير] وهو يورّم الكلى والكبد Ibn Zuhr ‖ ٣ يخلّ] يضرّ B ‖ ٥ بحح] بحة
ELU بحوحة O بحاح B ‖ ٦ وأشرّها] وشرّها ELU ‖ ١٤ الربو] الشهوة G G¹ ‖ ١٥ في تقوية النور
الباصر وينفع من ضعفه الكائن عن رطوبة وينفع من لسع العقرب. (٤٨) القطف له خاصّية om. ELO
‖ ١٦ الكبد] U¹ om. BELOU

yellow bile and is beneficial for the chest and lungs. Purslane has the special property of eliminating the craving[171] for clay and cures teeth that are set on edge.

(85) Asparagus [*Asparagus officinalis*] increases the sperm and has the special property of being beneficial for backache caused by phlegm and winds. When turnips[172] are cooked in fatty sheep meat, they increase the milk of a nursing mother and make it flow abundantly.

(86) Concerning taro [*Colocasia antiquorum* Schott.], al-Tamīmī contradicts the statement by Īsā ibn Māssa[173] that it is hot and dry and that it increases the libido. Al-Tamīmī states that it is hot and dry, produces black bile, and has no good in it. He says that saffron [*Crocus sativus* and var.] has the special property of stimulating the libido. Anise [*Pimpinella anisum*] has a similar effect; it also cleanses white humors from the uterus. Dill [*Anethum graveolens*] has the special property of being beneficial for hiccups arising from overfilling.

(87) He says: Peels of cucumber, especially those of the smaller[174] variety, if eaten, putrefy and produce a poisonous humor. Similarly, these small cucumbers [themselves] produce a poisonous humor if they are difficult to digest. If pregnant women constantly eat quinces, it improves the moral character of their children.

(88) He says: The special property of bananas [*Musa x paradisiaca*] is to obstruct the passages of the liver and vessels of the spleen through their viscosity and sweetness. Citron peels [*Citrus medica*] have the special property of being beneficial for sharp pain affecting the cardia of the stomach caused by the predominance and irritation of black bile. Hazelnuts have a special property to strengthen the jejunum and to avert harm from it.

(89) Hearts of date palms have a special property to extinguish and alleviate the boiling heat of blood. They are beneficial for bloody plague spots.

This is the end of the twentieth treatise.

الصفراوي نافع للصدر والرئة. وللرجلة خاصّية في قطع شهوة الطين وتبرئ من الضرس.

(٨٥) الهليون يزيد في المني وله خاصّية في النفع من وجع الظهر الكائن عن بلغم ورياح. السلجم إذا طبخ بلحم الضأن السمين زاد في لبن المراضع وأدرّه.

(٨٦) القلقاس أنكر التميمي ما ذكره فيه عيسى بن ماسّة من كونه حارًّا رطبا يزيد في الباه وقال التميمي إنّه حارّ يابس يولّد السوداء ولا خير فيه. وقال إنّ للزعفران خاصّية في تهييج شهوة الباه. وكذلك الأنيسون وهو ينقّي الرطوبات البيضاء من الأرحام وإنّ للشبثّ خاصّية في النفع من الفواق الكائن عن امتلاء.

(٨٧) وقال: قشر القثّاء وبخاصّة قشر الخيار إذا أُكلت عفنت وولّدت خلطا سمّيا وكذلك الخيار إذا عسر انهضامه ولّد خلطا سمّيا. وإذا أدمن الحوامل أكل السفرجل حسّن أخلاق أولادهنّ.

(٨٨) وقال: خاصّية الموز تسديد جداول الكبد وعروق الطحال بلزوجته وحلاوته. وخاصّية قشر الأترجّ النفع من الحزاز الكائن في فم المعدة من غلبة السوداء وهيجانه. وخاصّية البندق تقوية المعى الصائم ونفي الضرر عنه.

(٨٩) وقال: لجمّار النحل خاصّية في تطفئة الدم الحارّ الهائج وتسكينه وينفع من الطواعين الدموية.

تمّت المقالة العشرون.

١ شهوة] شوق EL | من] G¹ || ٢ النفع من] G¹ || ٣ وأدرّه] om. BELO U¹ || ٤ ماسّه] ماسويه BELO || ٥ ؛(يابس: قد) add. L | ٦ البيضاء] EOU ردي G¹ || ٧ في النفع] للنفع BELOU || ١٢ الحزاز] om. OU | الخفقان E | السوداء] المرّة السوداء BELOU | ١٤ الدم] om. ELOU || ١٥ الدموية] إنتهى كلام التميمي B هنا إنتهى كلام التميمي add. U || ١٦ تمّت المقالة العشرون] تمّت المقالة العشرين والحمد لله كثيرا E تمّت المقالة وعدد فصولها تسعة وثمانون فصلا L وقد كملت المقالة الكاف B كملت المقالة العشرين وعدد فصولها تسعة وثمانون فصلا O كملت المقالة الثانية عشر الحمد لله عدد فصولها تسعة وثمانين U

The Twenty-First Treatise

Containing aphorisms concerning drugs

(1) A treatment with nutriments that have therapeutic powers is better than a treatment with drugs that have alimentary powers. Be careful not to use pure drugs, unless you are forced to do so for some reason. When using drugs you should aspire to mix them with ingredients with alimentary powers that improve [their quality]. *In Hippocratis De alimento commentarius* 4.[1]

(2) Physicians have [always] used their skill to prepare drugs that promote health,[2] specifically those that have attenuating power, because this power opens the narrow passages, cleanses the viscous chymes that adhere to the vessels, and rarefies the thick moistures. But if a person uses them frequently, they make his blood watery or bilious and, with the passage of time, melancholic because these drugs, but for a few of them, heat and dry excessively. *De bonis [malisque] sucis.*[3]

بسم اللّٰه الرحمن الرحيم

ربّ يسّر

المقالة الحادية والعشرون

تشتمل على فصول تتعلّق بالأدوية

(١) العلاج بالأغذية التي فيها قوى دوائية أفضل من العلاج بالأدوية التي فيها قوى ٥

غذائية. فاحذر أن تستعمل الأدوية المحضة إلّا أن يضطرّك لها أمر من الأمور. فتستعملها

وتحرص أن تخلط بها ما يصلحها من الأشياء التي فيها قوى غذائية. في شرحه لثانية الغذاء.

(٢) احتال الأطبّاء في اتّخاذ الأدوية الصحّية وهي التي لها قوة ملطّفة لأنّ هذه القوة تفتح

المجاري الضيّقة وتجلو الكيموسات اللزجة المتعلّقة في العروق وتلطّف الرطوبات الغليظة

إلّا أنّ الإنسان إن أكثر استعمالها صيّرت الدم مائيا أو مرّيّا وعلى طول الزمان تصيّره سوداويا ١٠

لأنّ هذه الأدوية إلّا القليل منها تسخن إسخانا مفرطا وتجفّف. في مقالته في جودة الكيموس.

---

١ بسم اللّٰه الرحمن الرحيم ربّ يسّر [om. BELU ‖ ٣ الحادية والعشرون] الواحدة والعشرون L الثانية
عشر لجيس U

(3) Astringent[4] wine is beneficial in that[5] it stops all kinds of empty-ing. The best wine for someone suffering[6] from a hot disease is a watery one—that is, a thin white wine with no perceptible taste or flavor—because this wine does not have the harmful effects of water or wine. *In Hippocratis De acutorum morborum [victu] commentarius* 2.[7]

(4) Wine has the property of concocting humors whose concoction has not been completed. It stimulates micturition and perspiration and induces sleep. *De sanitate tuenda* 4.[8]

(5) The harmful effects of water are related to its coolness because water that is cold stays for a long time in the hypochondria and causes intestinal rumblings and flatulence and weakens and diminishes the strength of the stomach. This causes diminished digestion. And because of its coldness, it does not aid sizably in the transport of food. *De methodo [medendi]* 7.[9]

(6) The excellent qualities of the [different] kinds of beneficial wine are opposite to the afflictions arising from water. In addition, such wines produce beneficial blood, balance the temperament, concoct that which is retained in the stomach and vessels, increase the strength of the organs, and dispel the superfluities and[10] expel them with the excre-ment. *De methodo [medendi]* 7.

(7) Water does not alleviate cough and does not help expectoration; instead, it stimulates thirst, is transformed into bile, and weakens the body when drunk on an empty stomach. It increases the size of the liver and spleen when these are inflamed; it produces intestinal rumblings, floats in the stomach, and does not pass the excrements. It does not stimulate micturition, and its passage through the organs is slow because it is raw and uncooked. [Water] mixed with oxymel or the like is beneficial, however, because the other ingredient passes [the water] through the body and as a result moistens it; this also prevents its transformation [into bile]. *In Hippocratis De acutorum morborum [victu] commentarius* 2.[11]

(8) Barley gruel has a cleansing power that is so sufficient [on its own] that it does not need to be mixed with some hyssop [*Hyssopus officinalis* and var.]. If you want to increase its power, mix it with some [black] pepper [*Piper nigrum*]. There is no need to mix it with some honey unless you intend to cleanse the sides of the chest and the lungs. *De victu attenuante*.[12]

(٣) الخمر القابض ينفع جميع أنواع الاستفراغ ويقطعه وأصلح الخمور لمن به مرض حارّ الخمر المائي وهو الأبيض الرقيق الذي لا يتبيّن في طعمه ولا في رائحته كيفية. فإنّ هذا الشراب عادم مضارّ الماء ومضارّ الخمر. في شرحه لثالثة الأمراض الحادّة.

(٤) الخمر من شأنها أن تنضج الأخلاط التي لم يستكمل نضجها ويدرّ البول والعرق ويعين على النوم. رابعة تدبير الصحّة.

٥

(٥) مضارّ الماء منسوبة إلى برودته لأنّ الماء ببرودته صار يبطئ في ما دون الشراسيف زمانا طويلا ويحدث قراقرا ونفخا ويخمل قوة المعدة ويضعفها فيكون ذلك سببا لقلّة الاستمراء. ولبرودته لا يعين على نفوذ الطعام معونة ذات قدر. سابعة الحيلة.

(٦) فضائل أنواع الشراب المحمودة مضادّة للآفات الحادثة من الماء وفيها مع ذلك أنّها تولّد دما محمودا وتعدّل المزاج وتنضج ما هو محتقن في المعدة والعروق وتزيد في قوة الأعضاء وتبدرق الفضول وتسوقها إلى البراز. سابعة الحيلة.

١٠

(٧) الماء لا يسكن السعال ولا يعين على النفث ويهيّج العطش ويستحيل إلى المرار ويضعف الأبدان إذا شرب على خلاء جوف ويزيد في عظم الكبد والطحال إذا كان فيها تلهّب ويحدث قراقر ويطفو في المعدة ولا يحدر البراز ولا يدرّ البول ونفوذه في الأعضاء بطيء لأنّه نيء غير نضيج. وإنّما ينفع إذا اختلط بالسكنجبين أو بغيره لأنّ غيره ينفذه ويرطّب به البدن ويمنع من استحالته. في شرحه لثالثة الأمراض الحادّة.

١٥

(٨) كشك الشعير فيه من قوة الجلاء مقدار كاف حتّى أنّه ليس يحتاج أن يخلط فيه شيء من الزوفا. فإن أردت أن تزيد قوته فاخلط معه شيئا من الفلفل ولا تحتاج أن تخلط معه شيئا من العسل إلّا أن تقصد به قاصدا لتنقية نواحي الصدر والرئة. في مقالته في التدبير الملطّف.

---

(9) I have personally observed that barley has a cooling force, whether prepared as bread, groats, or *sawīq*.[13] Even[14] if its outer shell is not removed, the gruel prepared from it has a strong cleansing effect and, from another point of view, one does not suffer any harm from it. Because[15] barley groats have an effect opposite to that of lentils, a most excellent dish is produced when both ingredients are mixed together. *De alimentorum [facultatibus]* 1.

(10) The constant consumption of milk is harmful for the teeth and the gums and accelerates [the occurrence of] putrefaction and corrosion therein. Therefore, one should rinse one's mouth with diluted wine and honey thereafter. But sour milk is not harmful for the teeth, unless someone [who drinks it] has a cold temperament. And if the stomach is warmer than necessary, it is able to digest sour milk [well] and to derive some benefit from it, even if it has been cooled with snow. *De alimentorum facultatibus* 3.[16]

(11) The best [kind of] milk, after women's milk, is from animals whose nature is close to that of human beings, such as pigs, sheep, goats, and horses. Milk can be prepared by making solid,[17] smooth stones glowing hot after they have been washed, then extinguishing them in the milk, then boiling the milk so that most[18] of the moist, watery part disappears. When the milk is then taken from the fire and drunk, it alleviates dysentery and stops the diarrhea of[19] oily things. It is good for any biting tumor or ulcer that is dripping because of a surplus of sharp moistures. If instead of stones one uses an iron [object] that is free from rust, it is [even] better because it is somewhat astringent. *De [simplicium] medicamentorum [temperamentis ac facultatibus]* 10.[20]

(12) Milk has the property of changing and altering very rapidly, just like sperm. Therefore, in the case of milk, the best thing [to do], for someone who needs it, is to suck it from the breast. Women's milk is the best of all milks for those suffering from marasmus, and after it comes the milk of donkeys. *De methodo [medendi]* 7.[21]

(٩) الشعير نجد فيه عيانا قوة تبريد في ما يتّخذ منه من خبز أو كشك أو سويق ولو أنّ الشعير لم ينقشر عنه قشره الأعلى لكان الكشك المتّخذ منه أبلغ في الجلاء ولا يناله به مضرّة من وجه آخر. ولأنّ كشك الشعير مضادًا في قوته لقوة العدس صار متى خلطا جميعا تولّد بينهما غذاء هو أفضل الأغذية. أولى الأغذية.

(١٠) مداومة استعمال اللبن يضرّ الأسنان واللثة ويسرع إليها العفونة والتأكّل ولذلك ينبغي أن يتمضمض بعده بشراب ممزوج وعسل. وأمّا اللبن الحامض فإنّه لا يضرّ الأسنان إلّا أن يكون مزاجه باردا. والمعدة التي هي أسخن ممّا ينبغي تهضم اللبن الحامض وتنتفع به ولو برّد بالثلج. ثالثة الأغذية.

(١١) أفضل الألبان بعد ألبان النساء ألبان الحيوانات القريبة من طبيعة الإنسان كالخنازير والضأن والمعز والخيل. وإذا هيّئ اللبن بأن تحمى حجارة صمّ ملص بعد غسلها وتطفأ فيه ثمّ يطبخ اللبن طبخا تنقص به مائيته وأكثر رطوبته ثم ينزل من على النار ويستعمل سكّن استلاق البطن المفرط وقطع اختلاف الأشياء الدهنية واستعمله في كلّ ورم لذّاع أو قرحة سائلة من كثرة الرطوبات اللذّاعة. وإن استعمل مكان الحجارة الحديد النقي من الصداء كان أجود ليسير القبض الذي فيه. عاشرة الأدوية.

(١٢) من شأن اللبن أن يستحيل ويتغيّر في أسرع الأوقات بمنزلة المني ولهذا صار الأجود في اللبن أن يرضعه من يحتاج إليه من الثدي ولبن النساء أفضل الألبان كلّها للمذبولين وبعده لبن الأتن. سابعة الحيلة.

(13) The watery part of milk is a thinning substance, too, as well as stool softener. It is good to use it frequently, at[22] certain intervals. *De victu attenuante.*[23]

(14) The watery part of milk is better than all other things that relieve the bowels. I think that for this reason the ancient [physicians] used this drink whenever it was necessary to relieve the bowels. One should add enough honey to sweeten its taste so that someone who takes it enjoys it without feeling nauseated. And add as much salt to it as does not harm the sense of taste. If you want to cleanse the bowels in a stronger way, put more salt into it. *De alimentorum facultatibus* 3.[24]

(15) The most appropriate substance for expectorating the thick humors is hydromel and, for the viscous humors, oxymel. The second [best], after hydromel, is barley gruel, and after barley gruel, sweet wine. *In Hippocratis De acutorum morborum [victu] commentarius* 3.[25]

(16) Hydromel[26] boiled with absinthe wormwood is a remedy for passing the thin humors that are retained in the insides of the stomach. *De methodo [medendi]* 7.[27]

(17) If milk is added to honey, it is good for pains in the chest and lungs, but it is very harmful for the region of the liver and spleen. *De victu attenuante.*[28]

(18) Butter and honey mixed together are amazingly useful for expectoration from the lungs in patients with pneumonia or pleurisy. Moreover, it concocts [the humors]. If the butter is licked up alone, its concocting effect is greater but its support of expectoration is less. If butter and honey are mixed with bitter almonds [*Prunus amara*], [the mixture's] strength is greater in [helping] expectoration but is less in [helping] concoction. *De [simplicium] medicamentorum [temperamentis ac facultatibus]* 10.[29]

(١٣) ومائية اللبن فإنّها أيضا من الأشياء الملطّفة مع ما أنّها مليّنة للبطن واستعمالها مرارا كثيرة فيما بين مدّة طويلة صالح. في مقالته في التدبير الملطّف.

(١٤) ماء اللبن يفوق جميع الأشياء الأخر المطلقة للبطن. وأحسب أنّ بهذا السبب كانت القدماء تستعمل هذا الشراب في موضع الحاجة في إطلاق البطن. وينبغي أن يخلط معه من العسل بمقدار ما يعذب به طعمه ويستلذّه الشارب له من غير أن يغثي. ويخلط معه من الملح بمقدار ما لا يؤذي حاسّة المذاق. وإن أردت أن تطلق البطن أكثر فألق فيه ملحا أكثر. ثالثة الأغذية.

(١٥) أوفق الأشياء لنفث الأخلاط الغليظة ماء العسل وللأخلاط اللزجة السكنجبين والثاني بعد ماء العسل ماء الشعير وبعد ماء الشعير الشراب الحلو. في شرحه لثالثة الأمراض الحادّة.

(١٦) ماء العسل المطبوخ مع أفسنتين دواء يحدر ما في جرم المعدة محتقنا من الأخلاط الرقيقة. سابعة الحيلة.

(١٧) إن خلط اللبن بالعسل كان صالحا للأوجاع التي في الصدر والرئة ومن أضرّ الأشياء لما في الكبد والطحال. في مقالته في التدبير الملطّف.

(١٨) للزبد والعسل مخلوطان منفعة عجيبة من النفث الكائن من الرئة في أصحاب ذات الرئة وذات الجنب وهو مع ذلك ينضج. وإن لعق الزبد وحده كان إنضاجه أكثر ومعونته على النفث أقلّ. وإن خلط الزبد والعسل باللوز المرّ كانت قوته على النفث أكثر وعلى النضج أقلّ. عاشرة الأدوية.

٥

١٠

١٥

---

(19) Vinegar, in addition to the fineness of its parts, has a considerable repelling and hindering force. Therefore, the physicians did the
right thing to mix it with rose[30] oil and use it in the beginning of brain
diseases. If[31] several days of the illness had already passed, they mixed
thyme[32] [*Thymus serpyllum* and var.] with these two [ingredients] so that
it would have a heating effect as well as a refining [one] because[33] this
drug weakens on its way [through the body] and its strength is dissolved
because of the bones that hinder it. Therefore, in this case, we [also]
use castoreum,[34] although we do not use it for other inflamed tumors,
even if they are in the final stages of decline. But during the decline of
tumors in the region of the brain, this medication is most useful. *De
methodo [medendi]* 11.[35]

(20) Vinegar is harmful for the womb and the other nervous organs
because it is cold, thin, and sinks into them. *In Hippocratis De acutorum
morborum [victu] commentarius* 3.[36]

(21) Strongly acid oxymel either dries out the [superfluous] matters
and increases their viscosity and stickiness so that it becomes difficult
to expectorate them, or thins the thick, sticky matters that are retained
in the chest and lungs, so that they [start to] flow suddenly and abundantly and choke the patient so that he dies if his vigor is not strong.
Therefore, it should be used only if one has great strength. *De acutorum
morborum [victu] commentarius* 3.[37]

(22) Slightly acid oxymel moistens the mouth and palate, helps in
the expectoration of sputum, quenches thirst, and opens obstructions
occurring in the liver and spleen and cleanses them without harm. It
checks the bile resulting from the honey, dissolves the flatulent winds,
and stimulates micturition by opening the obstructions. It facilitates
the passing of superfluities and bile into the intestines without any
harm whatsoever, except that it abrades the intestines if constantly
used. *De acutorum morborum [victu] commentarius* 3.[38]

(١٩) الخلّ فيه مع لطافة أجزائه قوة دافعة مانعة ليست باليسيرة. وقد أصاب الأطبّاء في استعمالهم إيّاه في ابتداء علل الدماغ بعد أن يخلط معه دهن ورد. فإذا مضت للعلّة أيّام خلطوا مع هذين نمّام حتّى يسخن مع اللطافة لأنّ الدواء يضعف في طريقه وتنحلّ قوته بسبب العظم الحاجز ولهذا نستعمل في هذا الموضع الجندبادستر و إن كنّا لا نستعمله في سائر الأورام الحارّة ولو كانت في آخر الانحطاط. أمّا عند انحطاط أورام ما يلي الدماغ فهو أنفع شيئا. حادية عشر الحيلة.

(٢٠) الخلّ يضرّ بالرحم وسائر الأعضاء العصبية لبرده ولطافته وغوصه فيها. في شرحه لثالثة الأمراض الحادّة.

(٢١) السكنجبين الشديد الحموضة إمّا أن يجفّف الموادّ فيزيد في لزوجتها ولحوجها فيعصر نفثها و إمّا أن يقطع الموادّ الغليظة اللزجة المحتبسة في الصدر والرئة فتسيل الموادّ بغتة بكثرة فتخنق العليل و يموت إذا لم تكن القوة قوية. ولذلك لا ينبغي أن يستعمل إلّا مع القوة القوية. في شرحه لثالثة الأمراض الحادّة.

(٢٢) السكنجبين القليل الحموضة يرطّب الفم والحنك و يعين على نفث البصاق و يسكن العطش و يفتح السدد العارضة في الكبد والطحال و ينقّيها من غير أذى و يقمع المرار الحادث عن العسل و يحلّل الرياح النافخة و يدرّ البول بتفتيحه السدد و يسهل انحدار الفضول والمرار إلى الأمعاء وليس فيه مضرّة البتّة خلا سحجه للأمعاء إن أدمن. في شرحه لثالثة الأمراض الحادّة.

٣ خلطوا] خلط LO || ٤ العظم] الطعم G | G¹ || ٩-١٢ السكنجبين . . . الأمراض الحادّة] om. ELO || ١٠ اللزجة] G¹ || ١٣ البصاق] البزاق ELO

(23) The most acidic oxymel beverage has three[39] parts honey and one part vinegar. The sweetest oxymel has seven[40] parts honey and one part vinegar. It should be boiled until [the two parts] become one. Then the foam should be removed little by little. *De puero epileptico [consilium].*[41]

(24) We give oxymel to some patients to drink as a medicine, not as a food. Similarly, we give many patients hydromel and barley gruel as medicine, not as food. *De victus ratione in morbis acutis secundum Hippocratem.*[42]

(25) Oxymel is the most suitable of sweet things that are used for a thinning diet. In addition, it does not have bad chymes, is not harmful for the stomach, and has nothing at all bad in it. It is the most cutting, not only of foods but also of all medicines. If someone wants an extreme cutting and thinning effect on the thick, sticky, phlegmatic superfluity [in[43] the body], he should use squill wine and squill vinegar. *De victu attenuante.*[44]

(26) Ibn Zuhr states that the [ingestion of the] oxymel beverage with the juice of boiled eryngium [*Eryngium campestre*] every day on an empty stomach protects against pleurisy and tumors of all the internal organs, and that constant soft stools also protect against that. [He also says] that the potion prepared with the different kinds of sandalwood[45] is beneficial during times of epidemic [diseases].

(27) Oxymel, if used excessively, causes abrasion of the intestines, stimulates cough, and is harmful for the nervous organs. *De methodo [medendi]* 11.[46]

(28) To find a remedy that consists of thin parts and that is really absolutely cold may be impossible, because vinegar, which is thinner than all other cold things that we know and use as medications, has some warmth mixed with it, and we find that it has a drying effect.

(٢٣) أمّا شراب الخلّ والعسل فأثقف ما يكون منه ما كان عسله ثلاثة أجزاء وخلّه جزءا واحدا وأعذب ما يكون منه إذا كان عسله سبعة أجزاء وخلّه جزءا واحدا وينبغي أن يطبخ حتّى يتّحد وتنزع رغوته عنه أولا. في مقالته في صبي يصرع.

(٢٤) أمّا السكنجبين فقد نسقيه بعض المرضى على طريق الدواء لا على طريق الغذاء. وكذلك نسقي كثيرا من المرضى ماء العسل وماء الشعير على طريق الدواء لا على طريق الغذاء. في مقالته في تدبير الأمراض الحادّة.

(٢٥) السكنجبين أوفق الأشياء الحلوة التي تستعمل في التدبير الملطّف. مع هذا فليس برديء الكيموس ولا ضارّ للمعدة ولا فيه شيء رديء أصلا. وهو أشدّ تقطيعا ليس من الأغذية فقط لكنّ من الأدوية كلّها. وينبغي لمن أراد أن يبلغ غاية التقطيع والتلطيف للفضل الغليظ اللزج البلغمي أن يستعمل شراب العنصل وخلّ العنصل. في مقالته في التدبير الملطّف.

(٢٦) قال ابن زهر شراب السكنجبين بماء طبيخ القرصعنة كلّ يوم على الريق أمان من الشوص وأورام الأعضاء الباطنة كلّها ولين الطبع دائما أيضا أمان من ذلك. والشراب المتّخذ بأنواع الصندل نافع في الأوقات الوبائية.

(٢٧) السكنجبين إذا أفرط في استعماله يحدث في الأمعاء سحجا ويهيج السعال ويضرّ بالأعضاء العصبانية. حادية عشر الحيلة.

(٢٨) وجود دواء لطيف الأجزاء صادق البرودة محضها أمر عساء لا يمكن لأنّ الخلّ الذي هو ألطف من جميع ما نعرفه من الأشياء الباردة التي تداوى بها قد يخالطه شيء حارّ ونجده

١ فأثقف] فأوفق B || ٢ وأعذب . . . جزءا واحدا] om. G || ٣ يتّحد] يثخن L يحثر B || ١١ ابن] بن BLO | على الريق] G¹ || ١٢ أيضا] G¹ || ١٣ بأنواع] G² || ١٦ وجود . . . عاشرة الحيلة] om. G | عساه] عسر B عسر عساه L

Therefore, we mix enough cold water with it as to make it drinkable, and we use it for the diseases that need cooling and moistening. *De methodo [medendi]* 10.[47]

(29) We find a single medication having opposite effects, such as sorrel [*Rumex acetosa*], whose leaves relieve the bowels but whose seeds constipate. Similarly, a broth of cocks, snails, and cabbage juice relieves the bowels, but the meat [of cocks and snails] and the leaves [of the cabbage] constipate. Aloe and copper scales are astringent for moist wounds and strongly relieve the bowels. But cheese constipates the belly, while whey relieves the bowels. *De theriaca ad Pisonem.*[48]

(30) We find that [some] medications are beneficial for some organs of the body, such as agrimony [*Agrimonia eupatoria*], for it is clearly beneficial for the liver, and similarly, Chinese rhubarb [*Rheum palmatum* var. *tanguticum*]. Not every medication is beneficial for every person; rather, for each person there is a medication appropriate for him. *De theriaca ad Pisonem.*[49]

(31) The things that are most beneficial for the stomach are between bitter and astringent, such as the tendrils of the blackberry and those of the vine. All astringent things are beneficial for the stomach in most cases. *De victu attenuante.*[50]

(32) The best medicine[51] in each of its [different] kinds is neither[52] thin nor meager. Similarly, that which is thicker and fatter than the average amount is more deficient. Every [herb] for which the type-specific odor is very strong is the best. The same analogy applies to the taste [of herbs].[53] The excellence of compound medicines depends on the excellence of the simple ingredients therein. The difference between the two caused by their [different] preparation is small. *De antidotis* 1.[54]

يجفّف ولهذا نخلط معه من الماء البارد قدر ما يمكن شربه ونستعمله في الأمراض التي تحتاج إلى تبريد وترطيب. عاشرة الحيلة.

(٢٩) نجد الدواء الواحد يفعل أفعالا متضادّة كالحمّاض ورقه يسهل البطن وبزره يعقل وكذلك أمراق الديوك والحلزونات وماء الكرنب تطلق البطن وأجرامها تعقل والصبر وتوبال النحاس يقبضان الجراحات الرطبة و يسهلان البطن إسهالا كثيرا. والجبن يعقل البطن وماء الجبن يطلق البطن. في مقالته في الدرياق إلى قيصر.

(٣٠) نجد أدوية تنفع بعض أعضاء البدن كالغافت فإنّه ينفع الكبد منفعة بيّنة وكذلك الراوند الصيني. وليس كلّ دواء نافعا لكلّ إنسان بل لكلّ إنسان دواء من الأدوية موافق له. في مقالة الدرياق إلى قيصر.

(٣١) أنفع الأشياء للمعدة ما كان بين المرارة والقبض مثل قضبان شجرة العلّيق وقضبان الكرم وجميع الأشياء القابضة نافعة للمعدة في أكثر الأمر. في مقالته في التدبير الملطّف.

(٣٢) أفضل الأدوية في كلّ واحد من أجناسها ما كان ليس بمتشنّج ولا مهزول. وكذلك ما كان منها أغلظ وأسمن من المقدار المعتدل فهو أنقص وكلّ ما كانت رائحته التي تخصّ جنسه قوية جدّا فهو أفضل وهو القياس في الطعم. وفضيلة الأدوية المركّبة تكون عن فضيلة بسائطها. وأمّا الفصل بينهما بسبب صنعتهما فيسير. أولى الأدوية المقابلة للأدواء.

٦ الدرياق] الترياق BELOU ‖ ٨ بل لكلّ إنسان] om. L ‖ ٩ في مقالة الدرياق إلى قيصر] في مقالته تلك ELO | الدرياق] الترياق BU ‖ ١٢ أجناسها] أجناسه ELOU | بمتشنّج] بمشنّج Be, fol. 238a ELO | وكذلك] Be كأنّ | G١ أنضج] أنقص ‖ ١٣ أنقص] Be | وكلّ ما] وسائر الأدوية ما Be ‖ ١٤ وهو القياس في الطعم] وكذلك قد يدلّ الطعم على الأفضل من أنواع ذلك الدواء Be | عن] من B غير Be ‖ ١٤ عن] من B غير Be ‖ ١٥ بسائطها] الأدوية البسيطة ألتي ركبت منها Be | صنعتهما] صنعتها EL صناعتها B صناعتهما OU | المقابلة للأدواء] G١

(33) We should not use white hellebore [*Veratrum album*] in our times because of the bad [physical condition] of the people. Their bodies are full of phlegm; the hellebore attracts it, and the patient suffers from strangulation. Instead, we should use agaric [*Fomes officinalis*] and the like. This was mentioned by Asklepios in his commentary on [Hippocrates'] book on [fractures] and their setting.[55]

(34) Dried figs, if eaten together with walnuts and rue [*Ruta graveolens* and var.] before the ingestion of a fatal poison, help and protect against its harm. *De bonis [malisque] sucis.*[56]

(35) Milk, garlic, boiled wine, vinegar, and salt are beneficial against poisons or against [substances] similar to poisons developing in the body.[57] *In Hippocratis Epidemiarum librum 6 commentaria 6.*[58]

(36) Says Moses: He means that any of these [things] or any combination may be beneficial against a poison depending on the individual poison and the individual [bodily] condition.

(37) Capers whet a jaded appetite and cleanse that[59] which is in the stomach and belly and excrete it in the stools. They open obstructions in the liver and spleen and clean them, if the fruit is taken with vinegar and honey or with vinegar and oil before [the consumption of] all other foods. *De alimentorum [facultatibus] 2.*[60]

(38) Long pepper [*Piper longum*] has the property of dissolving thick, flatulent winds and to expel that which has coagulated[61] in the region of the stomach towards the lower abdomen and helps in the digestion of that which remains therein. This is something common to all sorts of pepper. *De sanitate tuenda 4.*[62]

(39) Garlic is one of the medicines that dissolve winds more than any other dissolving substance. It does not produce thirst and dissolves flatulence more than any other food. Therefore, I call it the theriac of the villagers. *De methodo [medendi] 12.*[63]

(٣٣) لا ينبغي أن نستعمل الخربق الأبيض في زماننا لكثرة شرّة الناس فأبدانهم مملوءة بلغم فيجذبه الخربق فيختنق المريض و إنّما نستعمل بدله الغاريقون ونحوه. ذكر هذا أسقليبيوس في شرحه لكتاب الجبر لبقراط.

(٣٤) التين اليابس إذا أُكل مع الجوز والسذاب قبل أخذ السمّ القاتل نفع وحفظ من الضرر. في مقالته في جودة الكيموس.

(٣٥) اللبن والثوم والخمر المغلّي والخلّ والملح ينفع من السموم أو ممّا يتولّد في الجسم مثل السموم. في السادسة من شرحه لسادسة أبيديميا.

(٣٦) قال موسى: يريد أنّ كلّ واحد من هذه قد ينفع السمّ وما يتركّب منها بحسب سمّ سمّ وحالة حالة.

(٣٧) الكبّر يحرّك الشهوة المقصّرة ويجلو ما في المعدة والبطن من البلغم ويخرجه بالبراز و يفتح سدد الكبد والطحال و ينقّيهما إذا استعملت هذه الثمرة مع خلّ وعسل أو خلّ وزيت قبل سائر الطعام كلّه. ثانية الأغذية.

(٣٨) الدار فلفل من شأنه تحلّل الرياح النافخة الغليظة و يدفع ما تجبّن في المعدة وما يليها إلى أسفل البطن و يعين على انهضام ما يتبقّى فيها. وهذا أمر يعمّ جميع أصناف الفلفل. رابعة تدبير الصحّة.

(٣٩) الثوم من الأدوية التي تحلّل الرياح أكثر من كلّ شيء يحلّلها ولا يعطش ويحلّ النفخ أكثر من جميع الأطعمة ولهذا أنا أسمّيه ترياق القرويين. ثانية عشر الحيلة.

١ فأبدانهم] أبدانهم EL لأنّ أبدانهم B || ٢ فيجذبه الحربق] G¹ || ٣ لبقراط] لابقراط BELO || ٧ أبيديميا] أفيديميا ELU || ١٣ تحلّل] أن يحلّل L أن يحلّل BELOU النافخة] om. LO || ١٦ ويحلّ] ويحلّل BELOU

(40) Obstructions and hard[64] tumors in the spleen require strong cutting, refining, and opening drugs. The skins of caper roots have the same effect on the spleen as absinthe wormwood on the liver, and rusty-back[65] fern [or hart's tongue fern] has the same effect on the spleen as agrimony on the liver. Caper with vinegar and honey is beneficial for both these organs. *De methodo [medendi]* 13.[66]

(41) Boiled melilot [*Melilotus officinalis*] has a concocting and astringent effect and is [thus] similar to saffron. *Mayāmir* 4.[67]

(42) Cinnamon [*Cinnamomum verum*] is a very fine drug; it opens the passages of the stomach, cleanses and attenuates the humors, and has a contrary effect on all the putrefactive[68] serous discharges by changing and dissolving them. Because of its pleasant aroma, it is beneficial for all diseases originating from bad humors; it is good for any putrefaction and counteracts any putrefactive force and restores it to a healthy state. Similarly, it is good for seropurulent discharges, fatal drugs, and animal poisons. After cinnamon, cassia [*Cinnamomum cassia*] (when it is first-rate) has this effect, and after cassia, the [whole][69] class of spices and aromatic herbs, such as nard, camel grass [*Cymbopogon schoenanthus*], lemon grass [*Cymbopogon martini*], and spignel [*Meum athamanticum*]. *Mayāmir* 8.[70]

(43) Aloe, although moderate, exerts an extremely contrary effect on someone affected by a hot, dry dyscrasia, but not by bad moistures. *Mayāmir* 8.[71]

(44) Absinthe wormwood has the property to cleanse, wash, and pass the bad humors retained in the cardia of the stomach, and to contract, strengthen, and fortify it. *Mayāmir* 8.[72]

(45) Bdellium [from *Commiphora mukul*] softens adequately, concocts, and, moreover, dissolves to a moderate degree. Resin from the terebinth tree has a potency similar to this one [bdellium] and, moreover, cleanses, purifies, and opens the narrow passages. These properties are needed for a weak liver. *Mayāmir* 8.[73]

(٤٠) سدد الطحال وأورامه الصلبة تحتاج إلى أدوية تقطع وتلطّف وتفتّح تقطيعا وتفتيحا قويا. وقشور أصول الكبّر للطحال بمنزلة الأفسنتين للكبد. والسقولوفندريون للطحال بمنزلة الغافت للكبد. والكبّر مع الخلّ والعسل ينفع هذين العضوين. ثالثة عشر الحيلة.

(٤١) إكليل الملك المطبوخ فيه مع الإنضاج قبض وهو مجانس للزعفران. رابعة الميامر.

٥

(٤٢) الدار صيني دواء لطيف جدّا يفتح مجاري المعدة ويجلو الأخلاط ويلطّفها ويضادّ الصديد المنتن كلّه بأن يغيّره ويحلّله ويطيب رائحته ينفع جميع العلل الحادثة عن الأخلاط الرديئة ويصلح كلّ عفونة ويضادّ كلّ قوة مفسدة عن الفساد ويردّها إلى الصلاح. وكذلك يصلح الصديد والأدوية القتّالة وسموم الحيوان. ومن بعد الدار صيني في ذلك السليخة متى كانت فائقة وبعد السليخة جنس الأفاويه والطيوب كالسنبل والإذخر وقصب الذريرة والمو. ثامنة الميامر.

١٠

(٤٣) الصبر وإن كان معتدلا فهو في غاية المضادّة لمن أصابه سوء مزاج حارّ يابس خلوا من رطوبات رديئة. ثامنة الميامر.

(٤٤) الأفسنتين من شأنه أن يجلو ويغسل ويحدر الأخلاط الرديئة المحتبسة في فم المعدة ويجمعه ويشدّه ويقوّيه. ثامنة الميامر.

(٤٥) المقل يليّن تليينا كافيا وينضج ويحلّل مع هذا تحليلا معتدلا. وصمغ البطم أيضا فيه قوة شبيهة بهذه القوة وهو مع هذا يجلو وينقّي ويفتح المجاري الضيّقة. وهذه الخصال تحتاج إليها الكبد الضعيفة. ثامنة الميامر.

١٥

(46) Indian valerian [*Nardostachys jatamansi*] has a considerable concocting strength for all cold diseases. Celtic spikenard [*Valeriana celtica*]
is inferior to it [regarding this property].

(47) Similarly, saffron is a drug well known for concocting unconcocted humors and diseases. *Mayāmir* 9.[74]

(48) All drugs[75] that free [the body from poisons] are of two kinds.
Some of them change and transform the poison or fatal poison, and others attract the poison and expel it from the body. Any fatal poison is
indeed evacuated by means of drugs that are applied externally, and
these attract the poison either through their heat or through their whole
substance. Similarly, [the drugs] that transform the poison and free [the
body] from it [do so] either through a contrary quality or through their
whole substance. *De [simplicium] medicamentorum [temperamentis ac facultati-
bus]* 5.[76]

(49) Concerning all drugs that free [the body from poisons], one
should take an amount that does not harm the body because the dose
is too large and that is not weaker than all the fatal drugs because the
dose is too small, for then the fatal drugs overpower the antidote. *De
[simplicium] medicamentorum [temperamentis ac facultatibus]* 5.[77]

(50) For stings or bites by [all kinds of] vermin, one should administer a dose from the great theriac that is slightly heavier than a hazelnut, with fifteen ounces of diluted wine, which should be nearly pure.[78]
And someone who undertakes long journeys should, prior to having his
meal, be administered a dose of one large bean with six ounces of hot
water as a protection against the harm [caused by the consumption] of
[bad] waters. *De antidotis* 1.[79]

(51) To heal [the effect of] poisons, one should take the theriac in a
dose of one hazelnut mixed with three spoonfuls of wine. For other illnesses the dose is different, and [the dose of] the fluids to be mixed with
it is different.[80] Just as this electuary is beneficial for afflictions happen-
ing to the body, so too it is beneficial for afflictions of the soul and counteracts black bile itself; it removes its substance just as it removes the

(٤٦) السنبل الهندي فيه من القوة المنضجة لجميع العلل الباردة أمر ليس بيسير والإقليطي دونه

(٤٧) وكذلك الزعفران دواء مشهور بإنضاج الأخلاط والعلل التي هي غير نضجة.
تاسعة الميامر.

(٤٨) جميع الأدوية المخلّصة صنفان: منها ما يغيّر السمّ والدواء القاتل ويحيله ومنها ما

يجذبه ويخرجه عن البدن. وكلّ سمّ قاتل إنّما يستفرغ بالأدوية التي توضع من خارج وهذه

تجذب السمّ إمّا بحرارتها وإمّا بجملة جوهرها. كذلك الذي يحيل السمّ ويخلّص منه إمّا

بمضادّة كيفية وإمّا بجملة الجوهر. خامسة الأدوية.

(٤٩) ينبغي أن يكون ما يناوله من جميع الأدوية المخلّصة مقدار لا يضرّ البدن بكثرته

ولا يعجز وينحل عن جميع الأدوية القتّالة لقلّته فتقهره. خامسة الأدوية.

(٥٠) يسقى من الدرياق الكبير للسع الهوامّ أرجح من مثقال بقليل مقدار البندقة بقدر

خمسة عشر أوقية من خمر ممزوجة قريبة من الصرف. ويسقى منه لمن يسافر أسفارا بعيدة

لدفع مضارّ المياه مقدار باقلاة عظيمة مع ستّة أواق ماء حارّ قبل تناوله الطعام. أولى الأدوية

المقابلة للأدواء.

(٥١) المأخوذ من الدرياق لشفاء السموم مقدار جلّوزة يداف بخمر قدر ثلاث ملاعق.

فأمّا لسائر الأسقام فالمقدار مختلف والمائعات التي تداف فيها مختلفة. وكما ينفع هذا

المعجون الآفات العارضة للبدن وكذلك قد ينفع آفات النفس أيضا ويقاوم المرّة السوداء

---

١ والإقليطي] والإفريطي L والإفليطي B والإطليقي O ‖ ويخلّص [G¹ ‖ ويخرج G ‖ ٧ وإمّا] أو
BELOU ‖ جوهرها] الجوهر BELOU ‖ ٩ جميع [G¹ ‖ القتّالة لقلّته فتقهره om. ELO ‖ ١٠ الدرياق]
الترياق BELOU ‖ ١٢ باقلاة] باقلي BELOU ‖ ١٤ الدرياق] الترياق BELOU ‖ ١٥ تداف] تذاب L

malignancy of animal poisons.[81] It may be drunk for the bite of a mad dog, but it may also be dissolved in rose oil [so that it becomes] like a salve and applied on the wound externally. And then this electuary is sufficient for freeing people from the plague.[82] *De theriaca ad Pisonem*.[83]

(52) A skilled physician informed me that once a fatal pestilential disease occurred in Italy,[84] and he recommended that the people take the theriac because no [other] drug was beneficial against this disease. And every one of those who suffered from this disease and who took the theriac benefited from it and was cured, but every one who did not take it perished. And whoever took it before the illness affected him was saved from falling ill from it. This is not surprising since this drug is capable of counteracting poisons. In general, in whatever illness other drugs are ineffective, this drug is amazingly beneficial. *De theriaca ad Pamphilianum*.[85]

(53) The snakes that are used for the [preparation of] the theriac are the least harmful [types of] vipers. But nevertheless one should cut off the head because it contains the poison and the tail because it contains the wastes of their nourishment. *De theriaca ad Pisonem*.[86]

(54) If those who are bitten by a crocodile put crocodile fat on the site of the bite, it heals immediately. I have seen this with my own eyes. And in the case of [a bite by] a weasel,[87] if one takes that animal and rubs the site of the bite with it, it heals immediately. The same applies to the bite of a viper: if one takes the viper, pounds it, and puts it on the site of the bite, it alleviates the pain little by little. *De theriaca ad Pisonem*.[88]

(55) When you cook vipers, be careful to have only a charcoal fire beneath them. Add new salt and fresh dill, not dried, to them. *De theriaca ad Pisonem*.[89]

نفسها ويذهب مادّتها كما يذهب بخبث سموم الهوامّ. ويشرب لعضّة الكَلْب الكَلِب ويحلّ بدهن الورد كالمرهم ويوضع على الجرح من خارج وهنا يكتفى بهذا المعجون في تخليص الإنسان من الوباء. في مقالته الترياق إلى قيصر.

(٥٢) حدّثني طبيب ماهر أنّه عرض مرّة في بلاد إيطاليا مرض وبائي قتّال فأشار عليهم بأخذ الترياق إذ كان كلّ دواء لم ينفع في تلك العلّة. وكلّ من استعمل الترياق ممّن أصابته تلك العلّة انتفع به وبرأ ومن لم يستعمله هلك ومن استعمله قبل حدوث العلّة تخلّص من الوقوع فيها. وليس هذا بعجب إذ كان هذا الدواء قادرا على مقاومة السموم. وبالجملة فأيّة علّة ضعفت عنها سائر الأدوية فإنّ هذا الدواء ينفع منها منفعة عجيبة. في مقالته في عمل الترياق.

(٥٣) الحيات المستعملة في الترياق أقلّ الأفاعي مضرّة. ومع ذلك تقطع روسها لأنّ فيها هو السمّ وأذنابها من أجل فضلات غذائها. في مقالة الترياق إلى قيصر.

(٥٤) الذين يعضّهم التمساح إذا وضعوا شحم التمساح على موضع العضّة شفى من ساعته وقد عاينت ذلك. وابن عرس إذا أخذت تلك الدابّة ودلكت بها عضّتها شفت من ساعتها. وكذلك نهشة الأفعى إذا أخذت ودقّت ووضعت على موضع النهشة سكّنت الألم قليلا قليلا. في مقالته في الترياق لقيصر.

(٥٥) طبخ الأفاعي إيّاك أن توقد تحتها إلّا بالفحم واجعل معها ملحا حديثا وشبثًا رطبا لا يابسا. في مقالة الترياق إلى قيصر.

١ مادّتها] بمادّتها BELOU | سموم الهوامّ] السموم L || ٢ وهنا يكتفى] وكنّا نكتفى ELOU وهنا نكتفى B || ٣ إلى قيصر] فصل ولست أشير عليك أن تسقي الترياق في وقت الصيف ولا في بلد حارّ ولا ينبغي أن يسقى الشابّ ولا المحرورون فإن نحن سقيناهم فالشيء اليسير منه ولا ينبغي أن يسقى منه الغلمان البتّة لأنّ قوة هذا الدواء أشدّ من قوة أبدانهم فلا يؤمن أن تحلّ أبدانهم سريعا. وقد قسر رجل ابنه وهو غلام على شرب هذا الدواء فحلّل بدنه وأطلق بطنه فمات الغلام من ليلته. في مقالة الترياق إلى قيصر add. G | ١١ الذين... لقيصر] om. G | ١٦ في مقالة الترياق إلى قيصر] في تلك المقالة ELO

(56) There are four tastes indicating heat:[90] sweetness, which is the least warming, then saltiness, then bitterness, and then sharpness, which is the strongest of them. There are four tastes indicating cold- ness: tastelessness, which is the least cooling, then sourness, then astringency, then acridity. An oily taste indicates an intermediate qual- ity between heat and cold and [also indicates] fineness of the substance. *De [simplicium] medicamentorum [temperamentis ac facultatibus]* 4.[91]

(57) An astringent [substance] cools and dries and therefore draws together, compresses, contracts, pushes[92] inwards, and thickens. A sour [substance] cuts, separates, refines, opens, cleanses, cools, and repels. A sharp [substance] cuts, separates, refines, opens, and cleanses just like a sour [substance], but it [also] warms, attracts, dissolves, and burns. A bitter [substance] opens and purifies the passages [and] cleanses, refines, and cuts the thick humors without notable heat. A tasteless [substance] has the property to thicken, draw and bring together, mortify, and stu- pefy. A salty [substance] collects, contracts, and dries the moisture with- out notable heat or cold. A sweet [substance] slackens, concocts, softens, and rarefies. An oily [substance] moistens, softens, and slackens. *De [sim- plicium] medicamentorum [temperamentis ac facultatibus]* 5.[93]

(58) Some biting remedies have a heating effect just like the sharp and bitter [remedies], and others have a cooling effect just as the sour [remedies do]. Biting includes these three tastes.[94] Remedies are mostly dissimilar in their mixtures; an individual remedy consists of different ingredients, and therefore we find different flavors when we taste it.[95] *De [simplicium] medicamentorum [temperamentis ac facultatibus]* 4.

(59) Anything that is clearly sharp and biting, according to its smell or taste or both, is hot and has cutting and refining power. Similarly, anything that has a pleasant smell, or that gives you the impression when you taste it that it is aromatic, has less heat than substances that bite. Anything[96] that has an alkaline or salty taste—most of such ingre- dients have refining power and soften the stools. Bitter things also have a refining power not less than that of alkaline and salty things. *De victu attenuante.*[97]

(٥٦) الطعوم الدالّة على الحرارة أربعة وهي الحلاوة أقلّها ثمّ الملوحة ثمّ المرارة ثمّ الحرافة أشدّها. والطعوم الدالّة على البرودة أربعة وهي التفاهة أقلّها ثمّ الحموضة ثمّ القبض ثمّ العفوصة. أمّا الطعم الدسم فهو يدلّ على اعتدال في كيفية بين الحرارة والبرودة وعلى لطافة الجوهر. رابعة الأدوية.

(٥٧) القابض يبرد ويجفّف ولذلك يجمع ويلزّز ويقبض ويدفع إلى داخل ويغلّظ. والحامض يقطع ويفرق ويلطّف ويفتح وينقّي ويبرد ويدفع. والحرّيف يقطع ويفرق ويلطّف ويفتح وينقّي مثل الحامض لكنّه يسخن ويجذب ويحلّل ويحرق. والمرّ يفتح وينقّي المجاري ويجلو ويلطّف ويقطع الأخلاط الغليظة من غير حرارة بيّنة. والمسيخ الطعم شأنه أن يغلّظ ويجمع ويكنز ويميت ويخدّر. والمالح يجمع ويشدّ ويجفّف وينشف الرطوبة من غير حرارة بيّنة أو برودة. والحلو يرخي وينضج ويليّن ويسخّف. والدسم يرطّب ويليّن ويرخي. خامسة الأدوية.

(٥٨) الأدوية اللذّاعة بعضها قوّتها حارّة كالحرّيف والمرّ وبعضها باردة كالحامض واللذع عامّ شامل لهذه الثلاث طعوم. والأدوية على الأمر الأكثر غير متساوية في امتزاجها بل الدواء الواحد مركّب من أجزاء مختلفة ولذلك نجد عند ذوقه أطعمة مختلفة. رابعة الأدوية.

(٥٩) كلّ ما يتبيّن من رائحته أو طعمه أو منهما جميعا أنّه حرّيف ملدّغ فهو حارّ وفيه قوة مقطّعة ملطّفة. وكذلك كلّ طيّب الرائحة أو يكون إذا طعمته يخيّل إليك أنّ فيه عطرية فهو أقلّ حرارة من الأشياء التي تلذع. وكلّ ما كان في طعمه بورقية أو ملوحة فإنّ أكثر ما هذه حاله فيه قوة ملطّفة وهو مليّن للبطن. وفي الأشياء المرّة أيضا قوة ملطّفة ليست بدون القوة التي في الأشياء البورقية والمالحة. في مقالته في التدبير الملطّف.

١ وهي الحلاوة] الحلاوة وهي ELO | ٢ التفاهة] التفيهة L | ٨ ويجلو] om. ELO | ١٠ ويسخّف] ويسرف B | ١٣ والأدوية] كلّها .add BELOU | ١٥ يتبيّن] بين G | تبين B

(60) All bitter substances have not only heating[98] [power], but also drying [power]. At times, some acrid, sharp substances have much moisture mixed with their heat. Therefore, we eat many things with these properties. *De [simplicium] medicamentorum [temperamentis ac facultatibus]* 4.[99]

(61) Drugs that cleanse without biting are similar to soup prepared from broad beans [*Vicia faba*], barley gruel, roasted flax seed [*Linum usitatissimum*], and[100] thickened juice prepared from dried figs. Concentrated grape juice has relieving power and is nourishing. It is one of the least biting substances. Greater than the cleansing [power] of these [substances] is [that of] resin from the terebinth tree, frankincense [*Boswellia carterii* and var.], and skimmed honey. Even more cleansing [power is found in] meal of bitter vetch [*Vicia ervilia*], lily[101] roots, and opopanax [*Opopanax chironium* Koch] roots. *Mayāmir* 7.[102]

(62) Drugs that really alleviate pains, whether the cause is a cold or hot humor or a cold or hot wind and whatever the consistency of the humor, are those drugs whose heat is like the heat of the body or that are hot in the first degree. In addition, their substance is so fine[103] that it rarefies, refines, concocts, and evacuates the concocted material and expels it through the pores. Therefore, these drugs should not have any astringency at all. *De [simplicium] medicamentorum [temperamentis ac facultatibus]* 5.[104]

(63) The temperament of the drug that helps against the development of pus and purulent matter is hot and moist, similar to the temperament of the body in which you want to concoct [these matters]. The most beneficial fomentation for this is lukewarm water and water mixed with oil. The most beneficial embrocation is lukewarm oil, and the most beneficial poultice is meal of wheat with water and oil. *De [simplicium] medicamentorum [temperamentis ac facultatibus]* 5.[105]

(64) The physicians apply the name "softening remedy" to that which softens hard bodies whose hardness was caused by cold, especially if moisture is retained in these bodies, as in the case of a hard tumor. These remedies do not have a strong heating effect and do not have so much dryness that they dissolve and slowly disperse what has become hard. These[106] kinds of remedies are always more heating than the temperament of the body from which the hardness is to be dissolved. Examples of such remedies are gum ammoniac [from *Dorema ammoniacum*], bdellium, liquid storax [oil of *Liquidambar orientalis*], solid[107] storax [*Styrax officinalis*], and some types of marrow and fat. *De [simplicium] medicamentorum [temperamentis ac facultatibus]* 5.[108]

(٦٠) جميع الأشياء المرّة هي مع حرارتها يابسة. أمّا الأشياء الحادّة الحرّيفة فقد يوجد في بعضها مرارا شتّى رطوبة كثيرة مخالطة لها مع حرارتها. ولذلك صرنا نأكل أشياء كثيرة بما هذه صفته. رابعة الأدوية.

(٦١) أدوية تجلو من غير لذع بمنزلة الحساء المتّخذ من الباقلّى وماء كشك الشعير وبزر كتّان المقلو والعقيد المتّخذ من التين اليابس. وأمّا عقيد العنب فقوته تطلق وتغذّي وهي من أبعد الأشياء عن التلذيع. وأكثر من هذه جلاء صمغ البطم والكندر والعسل المنزوع الرغوة. وأقوى من هذه جلاء دقيق الكرسنّة وأصول السوسن وأصول الجاوشير. سابعة الميامر.

(٦٢) الأدوية المسكّنة للأوجاع بالحقيقة كان سبب الوجع خلطا أو ريحا باردين أو حارّين بأيّ قوام كان الخلط هي الأدوية التي حرارتها كحرارة البدن أو حارّة في الأولى ويكون معها لطافة جوهر حتّى تسخّف وتلطّف وتنضج وتستفرغ ما نضج وتخرج من المسامّ ولذلك لا ينبغي أن يكون فيها قبض أصلا. خامسة الأدوية.

(٦٣) مزاج الدواء الذي يعين في توليد المدّة والقيح حارّ رطب شبيه بمزاج البدن الذي تريد أن تنضجه. وأنفع النطولات في ذلك الماء الفاتر والماء المخلوط مع الزيت. ومن الصبوبات الزيت المعتدل في حرارته ومن الأضمدة دقيق الحنطة مع الماء والزيت. خامسة الأدوية.

(٦٤) الأطبّاء يوقّعون اسم الدواء المليّن على ما يليّن الأجسام الصلبة التي قد صلبت من قبل البرودة لا سيّما إن كان في تلك الأجسام رطوبة محصورة بمنزلة التي في الورم الصلب وتلك أدوية لا تسخن إسخانا قويا وليست بكثيرة اليبس حتّى تحلّ ما انعقد وتحلّله أوّلا أوّلا. وهي أبدا أسخن من مزاج البدن الذي تحلّل صلابته بمنزلة الأشقّ والمقل وعسل اللبنى والميعة وبعض المخاخ والشحوم. خامسة الأدوية.

---

٣ بما | ممّا BELOU ‖ ٤ وماء | ومن ELO ‖ ١٤ خامسة الأدوية | في تلك المقالة ELO ‖ ١٨ وعسل اللبنى والميعة وبعض المخاخ والشحوم] om. B | والميعة] G[1] ‖ ١٩ المخاخ] المخاخ EL

(65) All strong diuretics, such as the seeds of the [different] types of celery, have a strong heating effect, [as well as] fennel, carrot,[109] wild carrot [*Daucus carota*] seed, Massilian hartwort, valerian[110] [possibly *Valeriana officinalis* and var.], spignel, sweet flag [*Acorus calamus*], and asarabacca [*Asarum europaeum*]. Stone-crushing remedies should have [only] a little heat so that they cut the stones by their fineness but do not make them more solid or dry them by their severe heat. Examples of such remedies are root of asparagus, root of blackberry, germander [*Teucrium polium*], Jew's[111] stone [*Lapis judaicus*], burned glass, and squill vinegar. *De [simplicium] medicamentorum [temperamentis ac facultatibus]* 5.[112]

(66) Drugs that stimulate the development of milk, menstruation, and micturition are all of them hot but differ in the degree of heat and the quality of their dryness [because[113] the type of drugs that do not dry and moderately heat stimulate the development of milk.] And the type of drugs that have a stronger[114] heating effect but not a strong drying effect stimulate menstruation. Both these types of drugs also stimulate micturition, and the type that has an [even] stronger heating effect than these and dries as well is also a stronger diuretic but does not stimulate menstruation nor the development of milk. Therefore, this last type alone is called "diuretic." *De [simplicium] medicamentorum [temperamentis ac facultatibus]* 5.[115]

(67) Says Moses: If someone makes himself remember that which is not necessary to remember, it causes a deficient remembrance even of the things that should be remembered. Therefore, I advise remembering [only] the natures of the drugs that are often used in any place, whose names are well known, and that are employed internally. I rely in all this on the book[116] [on drugs composed] by Ibn Wāfid because he is known for his skill and for his correct quotations from Galen and others. For some mineral drugs, I rely upon Ibn Sīnā.[117]

(٦٥) الأدوية المدرّة للبول إدرارا قويا كلّها حرارتها قوية بمنزلة بزور أنواع الكرفس والرازيانج والجزر والدوقوا والسساليوس والفو والمو والوجّ والأسارون. وأمّا المفتّتة للحصى فينبغي أن تكون قليلة الحرارة حتّى تقطع الحصى بلطافتها ولا تجمعه وتجفّفه بشدّة حرّها بمنزلة أصل الهليون وأصل العلّيق والجعدة وحجر اليهود والزجاج المحرق وخلّ العنصل. خامسة الأدوية.

(٦٦) الأدوية التي تنفع في توليد اللبن وإدرار الطمث وإدرار البول كلّها حارّة وتختلف في شدّة الحرارة وفي كيفية اليبوسة. وذلك أنّ الأدوية التي تسخن إسخانا معتدلا ولا تجفّف تجفيفا قويا تدرّ الطمث وكلا هذين الجنسين أيضا يدرّ البول والتي تسخن أكثر من هذا وتجفّف تدرّ أيضا البول أكثر ولا تدرّ الطمث ولا تولّد اللبن. ولذلك يخصّ هذا الجنس وحده باسم المدرّة للبول. خامسة الأدوية.

(٦٧) قال موسى: تكلّف حفظ ما ليس الحاجة ضرورية إلى حفظه توجب قلّة الحفظ للضروري. ولذلك أرشد إلى حفظ طبائع الأدوية الكثيرة الاستعمال في كلّ موضع المشهورة أسماؤها التي ترد داخل البدن. وأنا أعتمد في ذلك كلّه على كتاب ابن وافد إذ قد علم مهارته وصحّة حكايته عن جالينوس وغيره وفي بعض المعدنيات أعتمد على ابن سينا.

٥

١٠

---

١ حرارتها] G¹ || ٢ والجزر] وبزر الجزر BELOU | والسساليوس] والسفاليوس LO والساسليوس B والساساليوس E || ٤ والجعدة] وقصطرن add. ELO || ٦ في] من LO

(68) Of the drugs that are intermediate between heat and cold, three of them are dry in the second degree: namely, citron peel, mace,[118] and lentils; and three of them are dry in the first degree: namely, maidenhair [*Adiantum capillus-veneris*], asparagus, and olive oil. And three are moist in the first degree: sebesten [*Cordia myxa*], manna,[119] and Indian laburnum [*Cassia fistula*]. Gold is intermediate between these two opposites and is refining. In total [there are] ten.

(69)[120] There are twenty-seven drugs that are hot in the first degree and dry [in the first degree] and that are commonly used: rice [*Oryza sativa*], sarcocolla [gum resin of *Astragalus sarcocolla*], French lavender [*Lavendula stoechas*], melilot, camel grass, chamomile [*Matricaria chamomilla* and var. or *Anthemis nobilis* and var.], melissa [*Melissa officinalis*], silk, tamarisk [*Tamarix* spp.], cabbage, cauliflower [*Brassica oleracea*], coriander [*Coriandrum sativum*], ivy[121] [*Hedera helix*], sugar, cypress [*Cupressus sempervirens* and var.], resin from the sandarac tree [*Callitris quadrivalvis*], senna,[122] pistachio nuts, madder [*Rubia tinctorum* and var.], cardamom,[123] white lupine [*Lupinus albus*], marshmallow [*Althaea officinalis*], dates, agrimony, agaric, Jew's stone, and corundum.[124]

(70) There are eight commonly used drugs that are hot in the first degree and dry in the second [degree]: namely, absinthe wormwood, bitter vetch, clover dodder [*Cuscuta epithymum* Murr.], nard,[125] fern [*Aspidium filix-mas* and var.], peony [*Paeonia officinalis*], fumitory [*Fumaria officinalis*], and bush basil [*Ocimum minimum*].

(71) There are seven drugs that are hot in the first degree and intermediate between dryness and moisture or minimally dry: namely, flax seed, wheat, labdanum,[126] mahaleb[127] cherry [*Prunus mahaleb*], manna,[128] storax, and pine nut [*Pinus sp.* and var.].

(72)[129] There are nine commonly used drugs that are hot and moist in the first degree: namely, chickpeas [*Cicer arietinum* and var.], black-eyed peas [*Vigna sinensis* Endl and var.], almonds, borage [*Borago officinalis*], bananas, Jew's mallow [*Corchorus olitorius*], sesame, jujube [*Ziziphus jujuba* Mill.], and ṣeqāqul[130] [*Malabaila secacul*].

(٦٨) الأدوية المعتدلة بين الحرارة والبرودة منها يابسة في الثانية ثلاثة وهي قشر الأترجّ بسباسة عدس. ومنها يابسة في الأولى ثلاثة وهي كزبرة بزر هليون زيت. والرطبة في الأولى ثلاثة وهي سبستان ترنجبين خيار شنبر. والذهب معتدل بين المضادّين لطيف. الجملة عشرة.

(٦٩) الأدوية الحارّة في الأولى اليابسة فيها ممّا يكثر استعماله سبعة وعشرون دواء وهي أرزّ أنزروت أسطوخودوس إكليل الملك إذخر بابونج ترنجان حرير طرفاء كرنب قنّبيط كزبرة لبلاب سكّر سرو سندروس سنا فستق فوّة قاقلّة ترمس خطمي تمر غافت غاريقون حجر يهودي ياقوت.

(٧٠) وممّا يكثر استعماله من الحارّة في الأولى و يابسة في الثانية ثمانية أدوية وهي أفسنتين كرسنّة كشوث سنبل سرخس فاونيا شاهترج شاهسفرم.

(٧١) وممّا هو حارّ في الأولى ومعتدل بين اليبس والرطوبة أو قليل اليبس جدًّا سبعة أدوية وهي بزر كتّان حنطة لادن محلب منّ ميعة صنوبر.

(٧٢) الأدوية الحارّة الرطبة في الأولى ممّا يكثر استعماله تسعة وهي حمّص لوبيا لوز لسان الثور موز ملوخيا سمسم عنّاب شقاقل.

---

٢ كزبرة بزر هليون زيت. والرطبة في الأولى ثلاثة وهي [om. L || ٤ سبعة] ستّة G خمسة وعشرين ELOU || ٦ قاقلّة] قاقلّي ELU قاقولّى B || غافت] om. ELO || ٧ حجر يهودي ياقوت [om. ELO U¹ || ٨ وممّا] وما L || و يابسة] يابس G || ثمانية أدوية] G¹ || ٩ سرخس] كرفس EL || ١٠ وممّا] وما G || ١٣ شقاقل] S starts here

(73)[131] There are thirty-two commonly used drugs that are cold and dry in the first degree and are frequently used: namely, myrtle [*Myrtus communis*], lichen [*Alectoria usneoides*], gum Senegal [*Acacia senegal*], emblic myrobalan [*Phyllanthus emblica*], yellow (citrine) myrobalan [*Terminalia citrina* Roxb], Indian[132] and Chebulic [*Terminalia chebula* Retz] myrobalan, eryngium, broad beans, acorn, chestnut, soldier thistle [*Picnomon acarna* Coss.], coral,[133] roses, azarole [*Crataegus azarolus*], sorrel[134] (which is the same as wild beet), caltrop [*Tribulus terrestris* and var.], pear, goatsbeard [*Tragopogon pratensis* or *Tragopogon porrifolius*], mung[135] bean [green gram (*Vigna radiata* L.) or black gram (*Vigna mungo* L. or *Phaseolus mungo* L.)], the fruit of Christ's thorn jujube [*Zizyphus spina-christi*], blackberry, barley, thistle,[136] mulberry, apple, quince, sour pomegranate, vinegar, carob [*Ceratonia siliqua*], and willow[137] [*khilāf, Salix aegyptiaca*] (which is identical with *al-ṣafṣāf*).

(74)[138] There are ten drugs that are cold and moist in the first degree: namely, plum, spinach [*Spinacia oleracea*], violets [*Viola odorata*], endive [*Cichorium endivia* and var. or *Cichorium intybus*], nenuphar [*Nymphaea alba* and var. or *Nuphar lutea*], cherry [*Prunus avium* L.], orache, beet, mallow [*Malva silvestris*], and licorice [*Glycyrrhiza glabra*]. [Licorice] is lukewarm and slightly colder than our [bodies]; it is also moderately moist; its most beneficial part is the juice from its root.

(75)[139] There are thirty-four commonly used drugs that are hot and dry in the second degree: namely, Roman nettle [*Urtica pilulifera* and var.], basil[140] (which is the same as *al-rayḥān al-qaranfulī*),[141] terebinth tree, balsam of Mecca [*Commiphora opobalsamum*], nutmeg [*Myristica fragrans* Houtt.], germander, birthwort [*Aristolochia clematitis*], bitter ginger [*Zingiber zerumbet*], bitumen[142] of Judea (which is the same as *al-ḥumar*),[143] lac dye, turnip,[144] mastic [from *Pistacia lentiscus*], musk, ambergris, aloeswood [*Aquilaria agallocha* and var.], *falanja*,[145] [Chinese] rhubarb, jasmine [*Jasminum officinale* or *J. sambac*], dog rose [*Rosa canina*], narcissus,[146] gillyflower [*Cheiranthus cheiri*], rustyback fern [or hart's tongue fern, *sqūlūfandriyūn*] (which is the same as *al-ʿuqrubān*), colchicum [*Colchicum autumnale* and var.], white horehound [*Marrubium vulgare*], aloe, safflower, honey, hazelnut, carrot, borax, lapis lazuli, alum, salt, and rennet.

(٧٣) الأدوية الباردة اليابسة في الأولى الكثيرة الاستعمال إثنان وثلثون دواء وهي آس أشنة أقاقيا أملج هليلج أصفر هليلج هندي كابلي قرصعنة باقلّي بلّوط قسطل باذاورد بسد ورد زعرور حمّاض وهو السلق البرّي حسك كمّثراء لحية التيس ماش نبق علّيق شعير شكاعى توت تفّاح سفرجل رمّان حامض خلّ خروب خلاف وهو الصفصاف.

(٧٤) الأدوية الباردة الرطبة في الدرجة الأولى عشرة وهي إجّاص إسفاناخ بنفسج هندباء نيلوفر قراسيا قطف سلق خبّازى سوس وحرارته فاترة أبرد منا قليلا ورطوبته أيضا معتدلة وأنفع ما فيه عصارة أصله.

(٧٥) الأدوية الحارّة اليابسة في الثانية الكثيرة الاستعمال أربعة وثلثون دواء وهي أنجرة فرنجمشك وهو الريحان القرنفلي بطم بلسان جوز بوّا جعدة زراوند زرنباد كفر اليهود وهو الحمر لكّ لفت مصطكى مسك عنبر عود فلنجة راوند ياسمين نسرين نرجس خيري سقولوفندريون وهو العقربان سورنجان فراسيون صبر قرطم عسل جلّوز جزر بورق لازورد شبّ ملح أنافح.

١ إثنان وثلثون] خمسة وثلثون BELO || ٢ هليلج] om. ELOU G¹ | أصفر] زمرد لؤلؤ فضّة سادنة add. S | om. GS || ٦ منا] add. ELO غرا add. Ibn Wāfid || ٤ الصفصاف] del. U. زمرد لؤلؤ فضة شاذنة add. ELO زمرد لؤلؤ فضّة سادنة add. S | om. GS || ٦ منا] add. ELO غرا add. Ibn Wāfid || ٩ فرنجمشك وهو الريحان القرنفلي] برنجمشك وهو الحبق القرنفلي Ibn Wāfid | زرنباد] om. BELO | كفر] قفر BELO || ١١ بورق] بندق ELO

(76) There are six drugs that are hot in the second degree and dry in the first or in the beginning of the second degree: namely, the edible[147] nut [i.e., walnut], saffron, fenugreek[148] [*Trigonella foenum graecum*], frankincense, lily, and dried figs.

(77)[149] There are six drugs that are cold and dry in the second degree: namely, behen,[150] rocket, wild[151] senna [*Senna tora*] seed, fruit of the ash tree [*Fraxinus excelsior*], moghat[152] [root of *Glossostemon bruguieri* D.C., *mughādh*] (which is the same as *mughāth*), and coconut [*Cocos nucifera*].

(78)[153] There are twelve drugs that are cold and dry in the second degree: namely, barberry [*Berberis vulgaris*], flower of the wild pomegranate [*Punica granatum*], gum[154] tragacanth, waybread,[155] horned poppy [*Glaucium corniculatum* or *Glaucium flavum*], sumac [*Rhus coriaria*], boxthorn,[156] gallnut [of *Quercus sp.* and var.], black nightshade [*Solanum nigrum* and var.], gum arabic [*Acacia arabica*], rhubarb-currant [*Rheum ribes*], and fleawort [*Plantago psyllium*] seed. The latter is intermediate between moisture and dryness.

(79)[157] There are eleven drugs that are cold and moist in the second degree: namely, purple amaranth, melon[158] [*Cucumis melo*], cucumber, [the smaller[159] variety of] cucumber, watermelon, duckweed [*Lemna minor*], truffles, apricot [*Prunus armeniaca*], gourd[160] [pumpkin], lettuce, and peach [*Amygdalus persica*].

(٧٦) الأدوية الحارّة في الثانية ويبسها في الأولى أو في أوّل الثانية ستّة وهي الجوز المأكول
والزعفران والحلبة والكندر والسوسن والتين اليابس.

(٧٧) الأدوية الحارّة الرطبة في الثانية ستّة وهي بهمن جرجير حبّ القلقل لسان العصافير
مغاث وهو المغاث نارجيل.

(٧٨) الأدوية الباردة اليابسة في الثانية إثنا عشر وهي أميرباريس جلّنار كثيراء لسان
الحمل ماميثا سمّاق عوسج عفص عنب الثعلب صمغ عربي رياس بزر قطونا منها معتدلة
بين الرطوبة واليبوسة.

(٧٩) الأدوية الباردة والرطبة في الثانية أحد عشر وهي بقلة يمانية بطّيخ قثّاء خيار دلّاع
طحلب كمأة مشمش قرع خسّ خوخ.

٢ والحلبة] والجلّنار BGS || ٨ أحد عشر] om. L | بطّيخ] G¹

(80)[161] There are sixty-two commonly used drugs that are hot and dry in the third degree: namely, asafetida [gum resin of *Ferula assa-foetida*], opopanax, gum ammoniac, bdellium, sagapenum [gum resin of *Ferula szowitsiana* D.C. and var.], scammony, galbanum [gum resin of *Ferula galbaniflua*],[162] anise, harmal [*Peganum harmala*], cumin [*Cuminum cyminum* and var.], caraway [*Carum carvi*], fennel, dill, nigella [*Nigella sativa* and var.], wormwood[163] [*Artemisia* spp.], garlic, oregano,[164] mint [*Mentha*],[165] radish, squill, rue, black horehound [*Ballota nigra*], capers, celery, yellow amber [resin of *Populus nigra*] (which is dry in the first degree and Ibn[166] Sīnā says that it is [also] hot in the first degree), bishop's weed, savin, wild carrot seed, sweet flag, epithyme, common polypody [*Polypodium vulgare*], stavesacre [*Delphinium staphisagria*], colocynth, ivy-leaved morning glory [*Ipomoea nil* (L.) Roth], turpeth [*Operculina turpethum*], hellebore [*Helleborus* spp.], gentian [*Gentiana lutea*], hypericum [*Hypericum barbatum* or *H. crispum*], myrrh [*Commiphora myrrha*], bay laurel [*Laurus nobilis* and var.], seed of the ben oil tree [*Moringa arabica Pers.* and var.], asarabacca, hyssop [*Hyssopus officinalis*], artichoke [*Cynara scolymus*], turmeric [*Curcuma longa* and var.], celandine [*Chelidonium maius* and var.], centaury [*Centaurium erythraea* or *Centaurea centaurium*], wild caraway [*Lagoecia cuminoides* and var.], mūmiyā,[167] cinnamon, zarnab[168] (and[169] some say that this is the same as al-falanja), grape[170] ivy [*Rhoicissus rhomboidea*], lesser calamint,[171] cassia, costus [root of *Aucklandia costus*], clove [*Caryophyllus aromaticus*], galangal [*Alpinia galanga*], and leopard's bane [*Doronicum pardalianches*], cubeb [*Piper cubeba*], peppermint [*Mentha piperita* and var.], thyme [*Thymus serpyllum* and var.], and castoreum (the latter is dry in the second degree).

(81)[172] There are two drugs that are hot and moist in the third degree: namely, ginger [*Zingiber officinale*] and large elecampane [*Inula helenium* and var.].

(۸۰) الأدوية الحارّة اليابسة في الثالثة الكثيرة الاستعمال إثنان وستّون وهي حلتيت جاوشير أشّق مقل سكبينج سقمونيا قنّة أنيسون حرمل كمّون كراويا راز يانج شبثّ شونيز شيح ثوم صعتر فوذنج فجل عنصل سذاب مرّوية كبر كرفس كهرباء يابس في الأولى وقال ابن سينا إنّها حارّة في الأولى. نانخواه أبهل دوقوا وجّ أفتيمون بسفائح ميوبزج حنظل حبّ النيل تربد خربق جنطيانا هيوفاريقون مرّ غار حبّ بان أسارون زوفا حرشف كركم ماميران قنطور يون قردمانا موميا دار صيني زرنب وقيل إنّه الفلنجة حماما حاشا سليخة قسط قرنفل خولنجان درونج كبابة نعنع نمّام جندبادستر يابس في الثانية.

(۸۱) الأدوية الحارّة الرطبة في الثالثة إثنان: الزنجبيل والراسن وهو الزنجبيل الشامي

١ حلتيت جاوشير أشّق مقل سكبينج سقمونيا قنّة أنيسون] S¹ || ٢ قنّة] راتينج add. G¹ELO || ٣ مرّوية] مرّ L مرية S² مرارة om. B U || ٤ بسفائح] بسبائج BELU || ٥ تربد] U¹ | كركم] كرم L | كرفس] كرفس L¹

(82) There are two drugs that are hot in the third degree and moist in the first degree: namely, earth almonds[173] [*ḥabb al-zalam, Cyperus esculentus*] (which are also called *fulful al-sudān*), and thapsia[174] [*Thapsia garganica, tāfsiyā*] (which is the same as *al-yantūn*).[175]

(83)[176] There are nine drugs that are cold and dry in the third degree: namely, hemlock [*Conium maculatum*], henbane [*Hyoscyamus albus* var. *niger*], mandrake [*Mandragora officinarum*], camphor [*Cinnamomum camphora*], tabasheer,[177] areca nut [*Areca catechu*], sandalwood,[178] tamarind [*Tamarindus indica*], and dragon's[179] blood [*dam al-akhawayn*, red resin of *Dracaena draco*], which is called *al-qāṭir* and also *al-shayyān*.[180]

(84)[181] There are four drugs that are cold and moist in the third degree: namely, purslane, sempervivum [*Sempervivum arboreum*], fungi, and knotgrass[182] [*ʿaṣā al-rāʿī, Polygonum aviculare*], which is called *al-qaḍāb* in Egypt (it has a restraining effect that is good for inflammations and stops bleeding).

(85)[183] There are fourteen commonly used drugs that are hot and dry in the fourth degree: namely, pepper and long pepper (which is less dry than [pepper]), mustard, pellitory [root of *Anacyclus pyrethrum*], marking nut [*Semecarpus anacardium*], kundus,[184] mezereon[185] [*Daphne mesereum*], pepperweed[186] [*Lepidium latifolium*], garden cress, caper spurge [*Euphorbia lathyris*], cocculus indicus [seed of *Anamirta cocculus*], spurge[187] [*farbiyūn, Euphorbia resinifera* and var.] (which is the same as *al-tākūt*), leek[188] (which has varieties), and onion (which has varieties that contain moisture).

(86) Poppy[189] is cold and dry in the fourth degree. The total number of drugs whose degrees should be remembered because of their frequent use is two hundred and sixty-five.

(٨٢) والأدوية الحارّة في الثالثة ورطبة في الأولى إثنان: حبّ الزلِمِ ويسمّى فلفل السودان والتافسيا وهو الينتون.

(٨٣) الأدوية الباردة اليابسة في الثالثة تسعة وهي الشوكران البنج اليروح الكافور الطباشير الفوفل الصندل التمر هندي دم الأخوين ويسمّى القاطر ويسمّى الشيّان.

(٨٤) الأدوية الباردة الرطبة في الثالثة أربعة وهي الرجلة وحيّ العالِمِ والفطر وعصا الراعي وهو الذي يسمّى بمصر القضاب وفيه ردع جيّد للأورام الحارّة ويقطع الدم.

(٨٥) الأدوية الحارّة اليابسة في الرابعة الكثيرة الاستعمال أربعة عشر وهي فلفل ودار فلفل أقلّ يبسا منه خردل عاقرقرحا بلاذر كندس مازريون حرف شيطرج ماهوذانه ماهيزهرة فريبون وهو التاكوت والكرّاث وهو أنواع والبصل وهو أنواع وفيه رطوبة.

(٨٦) الخشخاش بارد يابس في الرابعة. جملة الأدوية التي تحفظ درجاتها لكثرة استعمالها مائتين خمسة وستّون.

٥

١٠

---

١ الزلِمِ] الشيلم L || ٣ الباردة] G¹ || ٨ ماهوذانه] ماهاذانه BO¹ || ١٠ تحفظ] يجب حفظ ELOU يجب تحفظها B | درجاتها] om. B

(87) Among the drugs that are not taken internally but that are commonly used externally, there are four that are intermediate between heat and cold: wax, litharge, cadmia, and lycium juice [*Rhamnus saxatilis*]—except that cadmia and lycium juice are drying in the second degree, litharge [only] dries slightly, and wax is also intermediate between moisture and dryness. Some of these drugs [that is, those commonly used externally] are cold in the first degree and dry in the second [degree]: namely, stibium, henna [*Lawsonia inermis*], and tutty. And some of these drugs are cold and dry in the second degree: [namely], ceruse and the different[190] kinds of earth. Lead is cold and moist in the second degree. The total number of these drugs is ten.

(88) There are six drugs that are not taken internally and that are hot and dry in the third degree—namely, pitch, pine resin [of *Pinus* sp. and var.], and vitriol[191] in its different types. Sometimes they are used internally in a small amount. Further, arsenic with its types, sal ammoniac, and burned copper. Sometimes these too are used internally in a small amount.

(89) Four of these drugs [that is, that are not taken internally] are hot and dry in the fourth degree: namely, verdigris, sulphur, tar [of conifers], which is sometimes used internally in a small amount, and animal biles. The total number of externally used drugs whose degrees should be remembered is twenty.

(90) The[192] color of natural bile is yellow, and this should be used in medical practice. Green bile is less hot because the cause of its greenness is the dominance of moisture over it. If yellow bile is burned, its color turns black. *De [simplicium] medicamentorum [temperamentis ac facultatibus]* 10.[193]

(٨٧) الأدوية التي لا ترد البدن وهي كثيرة الاستعمال من خارج منها معتدلة بين الحرّ
والبرد وهي أربعة: شمع ومرتك و إقليميا وحضض إلّا أنّ الإقليميا والحضض تجفّف في الثانية
والمرتك يجفّف قليلا والشمع معتدل أيضا بين الرطوبة واليبوسة. ومنها باردة في الأولى يابسة
في الثانية وهي الإثمد والحنّاء والتوتيا. ومنها باردة يابسة في الثانية: الإسفيداج والأطيان. أمّا
الرصاص فبارد رطب في الثانية. الجملة عشرة أدوية.

(٨٨) ومن التي لا ترد البدن وهي حارّة يابسة في الثالثة ستّة وهي الزفت والراتينج والزاج
على اختلاف أنواعه وقد يرد البدن قليلا والزرنيخ بنوعيه والنشادر والنحاس المحرق وقد
يرد البدن قليلا.

(٨٩) ومنها حارّة يابسة في الرابعة أربعة وهي الزنجار والكبريت والقطران وقد يرد
البدن قليلا ومرارات الحيوانات. جملة التي يجب حفظ درجاتها ممّا يستعمل من خارج
عشرون دواء.

(٩٠) لون المرّة الطبيعي أصفر وهو الذي ينبغي أن يستعمل في أعمال الطبّ. أمّا الخضراء
اللون فهي أقلّ حرارة لأنّ سبب خضرتها غلبة الرطوبة عليها. و إن احترقت المرّة الصفراء
صارت سوداء اللون. عاشرة الأدوية.

(91) The bile of a bull is stronger than that of any other land animal. Next in strength is the bile of a bear, and after a bear [the bile] of
a goat, and after a goat [the bile of] a sheep, and after a sheep [the bile
of] a swine. Therefore, the strength of [the swine's] bile is extremely
weak. *De [simplicium] medicamentorum [temperamentis ac facultatibus]* 10.[194]

The biles of all birds are sharp, biting, dry, and strong. The bile of[195]
chickens and cocks is stronger and more[196] proper in medical practice.
De [simplicium] medicamentorum [temperamentis ac facultatibus] 10.[197]

(92) I know from experience that when olive oil is applied to the
body while the oil is cold, it adheres to it and obstructs its pores, but
when it is applied while it is hot, it dissolves [residues] from [the body].
De methodo [medendi] 6.[198]

(93) If a wax salve that has been prepared with three[199] parts of
[rose][200] oil and one part of wax is[201] softened with cold water and a little
bit of vinegar and is actually made cold, it cools and moistens the bodily
part one wants to cool. If it becomes hot [while] on the body, it should be
replaced by another one. Similarly, if a *dabīqī*[202] cloth is moistened with
cold juices [that have been mixed] with *sawīq*[203] of barley and vinegar
and placed on the bodily parts, it cools them. *De methodo [medendi]* 10.[204]

(94) [Pains[205] of the eyes and ears caused by such a humor (that is,
thick and cold) and by flatulent wind during fevers should be soothed]
by applying a hot compress with common millet [*Panicum miliaceum*]
because it is a very light substance and, moreover, drying, while the
vapor developing therefrom is neither biting nor harmful. *De methodo
[medendi]* 12.[206]

(95) A poultice prepared from wheat meal and moderately cooked in
water and oil promotes quicker suppuration than a poultice prepared
from bread. One prepared from bread that was very well cooked after
having been soaked in water and oil is more effective in reducing [an
inflammation] because of the salt and yeast in the bread. [Even] more

(٩١) مرارة الثور الفحل أقوى من جميع مرارات الحيوان المشي وبعدها في القوة مرارة الدبّ وبعد الدبّ الماعز وبعد الماعز الضأن وبعد الضأن الخنزير فلذلك مرارته ضعيفة القوة جدًّا. عاشرة الأدوية.

مرارات الطيور كلّها حادّة لذّاعة يابسة قوية ومرارة الدجاج والديوك أقوى وأدخل في أعمال الطبّ. عاشرة الأدوية.

٥

(٩٢) إنّي قد بلوت من أمر الزيت أنّه متى أدني من البدن وهو بارد تشبّث به وسدّ مسامّه ومتى أدني منه وهو حارّ حلّل منه. سادسة الحيلة.

(٩٣) القيروطي المتّخذ بالزيت ثلاثة أجزاء وشمع جزء إذا دعك بالماء البارد ويسير خلّ وبرّد بالفعل فهو يبرّد ويرطّب العضو الذي تريد تبريده وإذا سخن على الجسم زال ويعمل آخر. وكذلك العصارات الباردة مع سويق الشعير وخلّ إذا بلّت فيها خرقة ديبقي وجعلت على الأعضاء برّدتها. عاشرة الحيلة.

١٠

(٩٤) استعمال التكميد بالجاورس لأنّه أخفّ الأشياء وهو مع هذا يابس والبخار المتولّد عنه غير لذّاع ولا مؤذي. ثانية عشر الحيلة.

(٩٥) الضماد المتّخذ بدقيق الحنطة المطبوخ بماء ودهن طبخا معتدلا أسرع تقييحا من الضماد المتّخذ من الخبز. والمتّخذ من الخبز المطبوخ بعد نقعه بماء ودهن طبخا كثيرا أبلغ تحليلا لما في الخبز من الملح والخمير. وأبلغ منه في منع التقييح الضماد المتّخذ من دقيق الشعير

١٥

effective than the latter in preventing suppuration is a poultice prepared from barley meal cooked in the water in which the root of marshmallow had been cooked. Hereafter this water was, together with oil, poured over the barley meal and very well cooked. *Ad Glauconem [de methodo medendi]* 2.[207]

(96) Al-Tamīmī[208] says in his [book entitled] *Al-murshid*: juice of the large elecampane in bees' honey prepared with spices and musk, which is called "the potion of angels," is beneficial for old people and for those suffering from [superfluous] moisture. It dissolves their superfluous moistures, it is beneficial for pains in the joints caused by cold, it strengthens the stomach and the heart, whets the appetite, and stimulates the libido. He further remarks there that cassia neutralizes the poison of the scorpion and of snakes and clearly helps against these, and that it strengthens the uterus of women if they apply it as a suppository or if they take a sitz bath with it. He also states there that *ungues odorati* [opercula of snail shells] are beneficial for hysterical suffocation and epilepsy both as a fumigation and as a drink in a dose of one *mithqāl*[209] [mixed] with apple juice. Similarly, quince[210] juice mixed with musk is extremely beneficial for hysterical suffocation and for palpitation of the heart.

This is the end of the twenty-first treatise, by the grace of God, praise be to Him.

المطبوخ بماء قد طبخ فيه أصل الخطمي ثمّ يلقى ذلك الماء والدهن مع دقيق الشعير و يطبخ طبخا كثيرا. ثانية أغلوقن.

(٩٦) قال التميمي في المرشد إنّ شراب الراسن بعسل النحل معمول بأفاو يه ومسك وهو الذي يقال له شراب الملائكة ينفع المشائخ والمرطوبين و يحلّل رطوباتهم الفضلية و ينفع من أوجاع المفاصل الباردة و يقوّي المعدة والقلب و ينبّه الشهوة و يبعث على الجماع. وقال هناك السليخة تبطّل سمّ العقرب والحيات وتنفع منهما نفعا بيّنا وتشدّ أرحام النساء حملا وجلوسا في مائه. وقال هناك: أظفار الطيب تنفع بخورا وسقيا لخنق الرحم والصرع وزن مثقال منه بشراب تفّاح. وكذلك الميبه الممسّك غاية ⟨النفع⟩ لخنق الرحم والخفقان.

تمّت المقالة الحادية وعشرون وللّه الحمد والمنّة.

---

٧ في مائه | om. GS | بخورا | ذرورا L || ٨ غاية ⟨النفع⟩ | טובה בתכלית NZ || ٩ تمّت المقالة الحادية وعشرون وللّه الحمد والمنّة] تمّت المقالة E تمّت المقالة والحمد للّه على ذلك وعدد فصولها أربعة وستّون فصلا L تمّت المقالة B تمّت المقالة الحادية وعشرون والحمد للّه وعدد فصولها أربعة وتسعون فصلا O تمّت المقالة الثالث عشر عدد فصولها أربعة وتسعون U | والمنّة] قال أبو بكر بن الصايغ ينبغي أن يزاد في رسم جالينوس للدواء أثر قوله ما (من O) غيّر أبداننا هذا القول بحيث يكتسبها فيه وعند ذلك يكون القول خاصّيا بالدواء غير فاضل ولا مقصّر فإنّه إن اجتز ينا (اختبرنا E) بقول ما غيّر البدن دخل في هذا القول السيف والنار والحجر و إن زدنا فيه ما له قوة على أن يكتسب شيئا يغيّر به أبداننا دخل فيه الفحم والمكاوي لأنّها بالقوة ذوات هيئات تغيّر بها البدن. وقال أيضا: الدواء المفرد هو النوع من الجوهر الذي من شأنه أن يكتسب من البدن هيأة يغيّره بها والمركّب هو كلّ ما ينقسم في وجوده إلى نوعين من الجواهر كلّ واحد منهما دواء يجري مجرى الدواء فالمفرد إنّما يعني به المفرد المادّة والمركّب إنّما يعني به المركّب المادّة والمفرد المادّة قد يكون مركّب القوى كالغار يقون والزاج. تمّ الكلام والحمد للّه add. ELO

Supplement

Critical comparison of the Arabic text with the
Hebrew translations and the translation into English

16.3: سدّة (obstruction): **N** has כאב לחכוך (pain because of itching), which is translated by **r** as "pain from a sore." **Z** translates correctly as סתימה (obstruction).

16.4: كمّية الدم إذا قلّت جدّا (when the quantity of blood greatly diminishes): **N** reads جدّا as غذاء and accordingly translates: כמות הדם כשימעט המזון. This is translated by **r** as "the quantity of blood (that lessens) with the diminution in food." **Z** reads جدّا as غذاء as well and translates accordingly: כמות הדם כשהמזון יהיה מעט.

16.10: صفحة (outside): **N** reads the Arabic as صفة and translates accordingly: תואר. This is translated by **r** as "appearance." **Z** translates the term as שטח.

16.12: على العانة والحالبين (to the pudenda and groins): **N** has corrupted the correct Hebrew transcription for العانة, namely, הענה as עונה and has the following version: על העונה והחולבים. This is translated by **r**, following **m**'s interpretation of both terms, as "on the breasts and genitals."

16.18: ملامسة (contact): **Z** reads the Arabic ملامسة as ممالسة and accordingly translates: חלקות (smoothness). **N** translates the term correctly as משוש.

16.19: انبثاق (bursting): Reading the Arabic انبثاق as احتناق, **Z** translates the word as חניקה (suffocation), while **N** translates the Arabic correctly as בתוק.

16.21: إذا كانت رباطاته مع عظم الصلب ضعيفة بالطبع (when the ligaments connecting the uterus with the spine are naturally weak): **N** translates this phrase as אם תהיה הנחתה עם הגודל קושי חולשת הטבע. It is clear that **N** has read Arabic عَظْم (bone) as عِظَم (magnitude) and misinterpreted Arabic صلب, which can mean both "hard" and "spine." **N**'s version is translated by **r** as "if its position and size render (the delivery) more labored and weaken [the woman's nature]." **Z** translates correctly as בהיות קשרי הרחם שעם עצם הגב חלושים בטבע.

16.24: فم المعدة إذا اعتلّ (the cardia of the stomach when it is affected by an illness): **N**, reading اعتلّ as اعتدل (to be balanced), translates the phrase as ישתוה. This term is corrupted as ישתנה. Following **N**, **r** translates the phrase as "alterations in the mouth of the stomach." **Z** reads the term as تعطّل (to be abolished) and translates it as יהיה מבוטל.

16.29: فإذا مات بلغ من انفتاحه (but if it [i.e., the fetus] dies, it [i.e., the os uteri] opens): Reading مات as the negative particle ما, **N** translates the sentence as וכשלא יגיע מהפתחו. This is translated by **r** as "If the opening does not . . ." **Z** translates the Arabic correctly as ובהיות העובר מת יפתח הרחם (When the fetus dies, the uterus opens).

16.38: اجتماع الدم في الثديين يدلّ على جنون سيحدث (The accumulation of blood in the breasts indicates that insanity will occur): Reading جنون as جنين, **N** translates the sentence as קבוץ הדם בשדיים יורה על שהעובר יתחדש. This is translated by **r** as "The gathering of blood in the breasts denotes that a fetus is developing." **Z** translates the term جنون correctly as שטות.

17.14: ثمّ يمسك قليلا (Then he should wait a little while): The correct version, ואחר ימנע מעט, is corrupted in **m** as ואחר ינוע מעט. This is translated by **r** as "then move a little." **Z** translates the Arabic correctly as ויעמד מעט.

17.19: ومن أرباب المرار (Some bilious persons): Reading the Arabic as ومن رباء المرّات, **N** translates the phrase as ומהרבות הפעמים, which **r** then translates as "It is very often the case." **Z** does not translate this section.

17.36: والفراش اللينّ (a soft bed): The correct translation, והמצע הרך, is corrupted in **m** as והתמצע הדרך. This corrupt version is translated by **r** as "pleasant walks." **Z** has the correct translation: והמטה הרכה.

17.39: العصب المنبثّ في فم المعدة (the nerves that spread in the cardia of the stomach): Reading المنبثّ as المنبت, **N** translates the phrase as העצב

הצומח בפי האסטומכה, which **r** renders as "the nerve which grows at the mouth of the stomach." **Z** translates the phrase as העצבים הנמצאים בפי האצטומכה (the nerves that are in the cardia of the stomach).

18.1: الأدوية الصحّية (drugs that promote health): Reading the Arabic as الأغذية الصحّية, **Z** translates it as המזונות הטובות והבריאות (good and healthy foods). **N** translates correctly: הרפואות המבריאות.

18.3: ينبغي أن تجرّد العناية (to pay attention): Reading the Arabic تجرّد as تجدّد, **N** translates the phrase as ראוי שתתחדש כוונתך. **Z** translates correctly: ראוי שתשים השגחתך.

18.12: نَفَس (respiration): **N** reads the Arabic as نَفْس and accordingly translates the word as נפש, which **r** reads as "soul." **Z** provides the correct translation: נשימה.

18.14: حركاته (his movements): This term is read as حرارته (his heat) by **ELOU**, and following this reading, **N** translates the term as חומו. However, **Z** follows the correct tradition represented by **BG** and translates it as תנועותיו (his movements).

19.11: كذلك من حمّ من استحصاف (So too someone who suffers from fever because of tightness of the skin): Reading the Arabic حمّ as حسّ, **N** translates this as ירגיש, and **r**, as "those who feel." This aphorism is missing in **Z**.

19.34: الشيء السارّ لها (that which gives it pleasure): Reading السارّ as السادّ, **N** translates the phrase as הדבר הסותם להם, and **r**, as "and produce an unpleasant situation" and in n. 46: "which closes them." **Z** translates the Arabic correctly: הדבר המשמח להם.

20.18: بكدّ (with trouble): Reading the Arabic as بكثر, **N** translates the phrase as פעמים רבות, and **r**, as "quite often." **Z** translates the phrase correctly: בעמל.

20.54: تمر (dates): Reading the Arabic as ثمر (fruits), **Z** translates the term as פירות. **N** translates it correctly: תמרים.

20.68: وتخصّب (and fattens): Reading the Arabic as وتكسّب, **Z** translates the word as ויקנה. **N** translates it correctly: ומשמין.

20.84: ضرس (teeth that are set on edge): **N** translates the Arabic wrongly as שלשול הדם מן המעיים, which is translated by **r** as "diarrheal bleeding from the intestines." **Z** translates the phrase correctly: קיהות השניים.

21.2: اتّخاذ (preparation): **N** translates the Arabic wrongly as לספר, and **r** translates the term as "to describe." **Z** translates it correctly: לקחת.

21.6: براز (excrements): Possibly reading the Arabic as بارز, **N** translates the word as לצאת לחוץ, and **r**, as "outside." **Z** has the correct version: רעי.

21.10: لِثّة (gums): **N** translates the term incorrectly as לסתות (jaws), while **Z** translates it correctly: חניכיים.

21.11: اختلاف (diarrhea): The Arabic term has the general meaning of "difference" and the specific, medical meaning of "diarrhea." On the basis of its general meaning, **Z** translates the term as שינוי (change). **N** translates it correctly: שלשול.

21.14: ماء اللبن . . . هذا الشراب (The watery part of milk . . . this drink): It is clear that in this context the Arabic شراب means "drink." Accordingly, **Z** translates it as משקה. However, **N** wrongly translates it as יין.

21.17: أوجاع (pains): **Z** reads the Arabic as أخلاط and translates the word as ליחות. **N** correctly translates it as כאבים.

21.23: أثقف (most acid): **N** probably reads the Arabic as اتّفق, and, accordingly, translates it as יזדמן, which **r** then translates as "occasionally." **Z** follows **B**: أوفق, and translates the Arabic as הטוב (the best).

21.31: مرارة (bitterness): Reading the Arabic as حرارة, **Z** translates it as חמימות (heat). **N** translates the term correctly: מרירות.

21.57: المسك الطعم (A tasteless [substance]): **Z** reads the Arabic as الممسك الطعام and accordingly translates it as מחזיק המזון. **N** translates the term correctly as התפל הטעם, which **r** then translates as "a tasteless substance."

21.91: دبّ (bear): Reading the Arabic as ذِبّ, **Z** translates the word as זאב (wolf), while **N** translates it correctly: דוב.

21.93: تقيّح (suppuration): Reading the Arabic as تفتيح, **Z** translates the term as פותח. **N** translates it correctly: להביא מוגלא.

Notes to the English Translation

The Sixteenth Treatise

1. The authenticity of this work is uncertain; it is mentioned in Ibn Abī Uṣaybiʿah, ʿUyūn al-anbāʾ, 149, but not by Ḥunayn ibn Isḥāq. Cf. Meyerhof, "Über echte und unechte Schriften Galens," 542, no. 56; and Ullmann, "Zwei spätantike Kommentare." See also Bos's introduction to Maimonides, *Medical Aphorisms* (ed. and trans. Bos), 1:xxi. For the quotations from this treatise, see the introduction to this volume.

2. "water mint": Cf. Galen, *De curandi ratione per venae sectionem* 18 (ed. Kühn, 11:304): καλαμίνθη (mint). For its three varieties, see Dioscurides, *Pedanii Dioscuridis Anazarbei* 3.35 (ed. Wellmann, 2:46–48); *Pedanios Dioskurides aus Anazarbos* 3.37 (ed. and trans. Berendes, 287–88); and *Dioscurides triumphans* 3.35 (ed. and trans. Dietrich, 2:382–83).

3. "cultivated mint": Perhaps peppermint (*Mentha piperita*). For the problematic identification of this species of mint, see Dioscurides, *Dioscurides triumphans* 3.34 (ed. and trans. Dietrich, 2:381). Galen, *De curandi ratione per venae sectionem* 18 (ed. Kühn, 11:304), reads γλήχων (pennyroyal, *Mentha pulegium*).

4. Galen, *De curandi ratione per venae sectionem* 18 (ed. Kühn, 11:304), remarks that it should be applied in the same way as the other remedies mentioned before.

5. "hiera" (from Greek ἱερά): Name used for a number of compound medicines; see Ullmann, *Medizin im Islam*, 296. The most common is hiera picra, with aloe as the main component; see Galen, *De curandi ratione per venae sectionem* 18 (ed. Kühn, 11:304): "the so-called *pikron* remedy consisting of 100 drachmas of aloe and 6 drachmas of other drugs."

6. Galen, *De curandi ratione per venae sectionem* 18 (ed. Kühn, 11:303–4). For the Arabic translation of Galen's *De venae sectione*, see Steinschneider, "Griechische Ärzte," 289, no. 45; and Ḥunayn ibn Isḥāq, *Über syrische und arabische Galen-Übersetzungen* (ed. Bergsträsser, no. 71d).

7. See note 1.

8. "organ" (ʾāla): Namely, the vessels and uterus. Today we do not use this term when referring to vessels; see Savage-Smith, ed. and trans., in Galen, "Nerves, Veins and Arteries," 43.

9. "mention": "mean" in **BELOU.**

10. See the introduction to this volume.

11. "heaviness of the body": Not mentioned in Galen, *De locis affectis* 6.5 (ed. Kühn, 8:435).

12. "roots of the eyes": Cf. Galen, *De locis affectis* 6.5 (ed. Kühn, 8:435): τὰς τῶν ὀφθαλμῶν βάσεις.

13. "a dark, reddish urine": Lit. "urine with a color mixed from darkness and redness."

14. "flow of milk from the breasts": Not in Galen, *De locis affectis* 6.5 (ed. Kühn, 8:435).

15. "in the hollow of the groin": Cf. Galen, *De locis affectis* 6.5 (ed. Kühn, 8:434): κατὰ τὸν κενεῶνα.

16. Galen, *De locis affectis* 6.5 (ed. Kühn, 8:434–35).

17. "a bad complexion": Cf. Galen, *De locis affectis* 6.5 (ed. Kühn, 8:435): ἄχροιαι (paleness).

18. Galen, *De locis affectis* 6.5 (ed. Kühn, 8:435).

19. "the illness called *nazf* [female flux]": Cf. Galen, *De locis affectis* 6.5 (ed. Kühn, 8:436): ὁ καλούμενος ῥοῦς γυναικεῖος, and Ullmann, *Wörterbuch zu griechisch-arabischen Übersetzungen*, 592. This illness is now called *whites* (leucorrhoea).

20. Galen, *De locis affectis* 6.5 (ed. Kühn, 8:436).

21. Galen, *In Hippocratis Epidemiarum librum 6 commentaria* 8 (CMG 5.10.2.2; ed. Wenkebach and trans. Pfaff, 507, lines 11–13, 17–21; Latin in Deller, trans., "Exzerpta aus Epidemienkommentaren," 543, no. 113).

22. See note 1.

23. I.e., the ovaries.

24. Galen, *On Semen* (ed. and trans. De Lacy, p. 188, line 1–p. 190, line 18).

25. Cf. Maimonides, *Commentary on Hippocrates' Aphorisms* 5.50 (ed. and trans. Bos, forthcoming): "Says Hippocrates: If you want to stop the menstrual bleeding of a woman, apply the largest available cupping glass to each of her breasts. Says the commentator: This is clear because it attracts the blood to the opposite side."

26. For hysterical suffocation—a displacement of the womb whereby it comes into sympathy with the upper parts of the body, causing suffocation and sensory disturbances—see aphorisms 16.15–17 below. See also Ibn al-Jazzār, *On Sexual Diseases* 11 (ed. and trans. Bos, 153–60 [Arabic], 274–76 [English]).

27. "and sweet-smelling medicines . . . her uterus": Cf. Galen, *Ad Glauconem de medendi methodo* 1.15 (ed. Kühn, 11:54): ". . . and sweet-smelling medicines near her uterus. One should also apply medicines with slackening and heating properties."

28. Galen, *Ad Glauconem de medendi methodo* 1.15 (ed. Kühn, 11:54).

29. Galen, *De methodo medendi* 13.19 (ed. Kühn, 10:926); translation by Johnston and Horsley, *Method of Medicine*, 3:397: "And if we wish to set in motion the menstrual flow, we place the cupping glass on the pubes and the inguinal glands."

30. "Then you may also apply cupping glasses to both ankles": This advice does not appear in Galen, *De curandi ratione per venae sectionem* 18 (ed. Kühn, 11:303). See the introduction to this volume.

31. Galen, *De curandi ratione per venae sectionem* 18 (ed. Kühn, 11:303).

32. See note 1.

33. See note 1.

34. See note 1.

35. Cf. Galen, *De locis affectis* 6.5 (ed. Kühn, 8:418–21).

36. "Because of the afflictions . . . her uterus had been pulled up": Lit. "Because of the afflictions she suffered from as a result of hysterical suffocation and because of the information from her midwife who told me that her uterus had been pulled up." Cf. Galen, *De locis affectis* 6.5 (ed. Kühn, 8:420): "Since besides some other afflictions, she suffered from nervous tension, when her midwife told me that her uterus had been pulled up"; and **W**: "And because of the other afflictions that happened to her, for the midwife told [me] that her uterus had been pulled up."

37. Galen, *De locis affectis* 6.5 (ed. Kühn, 8:420). Nathan's Hebrew translation of this text is quoted by the MaHaRShaKh (Rabbi Solomon ben Abraham ha-Kohen), who lived in Thessaloniki in the second half of the sixteenth century, in his *Sheʾelot u-Teshuvot*, no. 105.

38. Galen, *In Hippocratis Aphorismos commentarius* 5.60 (ed. Kühn, 17B:859).

39. Galen, *De locis affectis* 6.5 (ed. Kühn, 8:436). Cf. Anastassiou and Irmer, eds., *Testimonien zum Corpus Hippocraticum*, pt. 2, 2:97 (Hippocrates, *Aphorismes* 5.38 [ed. and trans. Littré, 4:544, lines 11–13 (Greek text), 545 (French translation)]).

40. See note 1.

41. Galen, *On the Natural Faculties* 3.3 (trans. Brock, 234–35).

42. Galen, *Ad Glauconem de methodo medendi* 2.12 (ed. Kühn, 11:139).

43. Cf. Galen, *De symptomatum causis* 1.7 (ed. Kühn, 7:133–34). Galen's *De morborum causis et symptomatibus* consists of six books: *De morborum differentiis*, *De causis morborum liber*, *De symptomatum differentiis liber*, and *De symptomatum causis* 1–3 (see Ullmann, *Medizin im Islam*, 42, no. 22). For the phenomenon of craving bad food, called κίσσα (*pica*) in ancient sources, see Ibn al-Jazzār, *On Sexual Diseases* 15 (ed. and trans. Bos, 180–89 [Arabic], 285–88 [English]).

44. "symptom": Lit. "illness."

45. Galen, *De locis affectis* 5.6 (ed. Kühn, 8:343).

46. Galen, *De locis affectis* 6.5 (ed. Kühn, 8:437).

47. Galen, *De locis affectis* 6.5 (ed. Kühn, 8:437). Cf. Anastassiou and Irmer, eds., *Testimonien zum Corpus Hippocraticum*, pt. 2, 2:97 (Hippocrates, *Aphorismes* 5.38 [ed. and trans. Littré, 4:544, lines 11–13 (Greek), 545 (French)]); and Maimonides, *Commentary on Hippocrates' Aphorisms* 5.37 (ed. and trans. Bos, forthcoming): "Says Hippocrates: if the breasts of a pregnant woman suddenly become thin, she will miscarry. Says the commentator: The interrelationship between the breasts and the uterus is well known. When [the breasts] become thin, it indicates that [only] a small amount of food reaches them. If the nutrition that reaches the uterus also decreases, the fetus is aborted."

48. "openings of the vessels": Cf. Galen, *De locis affectis* 6.5 (ed. Kühn, 8:437): κοτυληδόνας; English translation by Siegel in *Galen on the Affected Parts*, 192: "cotyledons [of the placenta]." Also cf. Liddell and Scott, *Greek-English Lexicon*, 9th ed., s.v. κοτυλήδων: "*cotyledons*, foetal and uterine vascular connexions"; and Ullmann, *Wörterbuch zu griechisch-arabischen Übersetzungen: Supplement*, 1:585–86.

49. Galen, *De locis affectis* 6.5 (ed. Kühn, 8:437). Cf. Anastassiou and Irmer, eds., *Testimonien zum Corpus Hippocraticum*, pt. 2, 2:97 (Hippocrates, *Aphorismes* 5.38 [ed. and trans. Littré, 4:544, lines 11–13 (Greek), 545 (French)]).

50. Galen, *De pulsibus libellus ad tirones* 9 (ed. Kühn, 8:466). For the Arabic name of this treatise, see Ullmann, *Medizin im Islam*, 44, no. 32.

51. Galen, *On the Natural Faculties* 3.3 (trans. Brock, 234–37).

52. See note 1.

53. "the formative and growth-promoting faculty": Galen, *De atra bile* 8 (ed. Kühn, 5:137; ed. Boer, 88, lines 13–15), speaks about the nature that forms and promotes the growth of the fetus.

54. Galen, *De atra bile* 8 (ed. Kühn, 5:137–38; ed. Boer, 88, lines 13–17).

55. Pseudo-Galen, *In Hippocratis De alimento commentarius* 4.20 (ed. Kühn 15:407–8). The text of this commentary as edited by Kühn is a Renaissance forgery.

56. Galen, *In Hippocratis Epidemiarum librum 2 commentaria* 2 (CMG 10.5.1; ed. Wenkebach and trans. Pfaff, 231, lines 11–14; Latin in Deller, trans., "Exzerpta aus Epidemienkommentaren," 524, no. 21).

57. "She should be given fluid-promoting food": Lit. "she should be nourished and moistened."

58. Galen, *In Hippocratis Epidemiarum librum 2 commentaria* 6 (CMG 10.5.1; ed. Wenkebach and trans. Pfaff, 366, lines 14–15, 29–38; Latin in Deller, trans., "Exzerpta aus Epidemienkommentaren," 524, no. 21).

59. "If the milk . . . illness will occur" Cf. **ELOU**: لِرْ يستحكم. Also cf. Pseudo-Galen, *In Hippocratis De alimento commentarius* 4.8 (ed. Kühn, 15:394): "Milk of a bad quality is either thick or watery or serous or livid." Cf. Soranus, *Gynaeciorum* (ed. Ilberg 2:13); English translation by Temkin in *Soranus' Gynecology*, 95: "For free-running, thin, and watery milk is not nutritious and is apt to disturb the bowels; whereas thick and caseous milk is hard to digest and [. . .] it blocks up the ducts."

60. See note 1.

61. Cf. Hippocrates, *Epidemics* 2.6 (ed. and trans. Smith, 83, no. 18): ἢν στερεώτεροι ἔωσιν οἱ τιτθοί.

62. Galen, *In Hippocratis Epidemiarum librum 2 commentaria* 6 (CMG 10.5.1; ed. Wenkebach and trans. Pfaff, 387, lines 6–20; Latin in Deller, trans., "Exzerpta aus Epidemienkommentaren," 527, no. 33). See also Maimonides, *Commentary on Hippocrates' Aphorisms* 5.52 (ed. and trans. Bos, forthcoming): "Says Hippocrates: If milk flows from the breasts of a pregnant woman, it indicates that the [fetus] is weak, but if the breasts are firm, it indicates that the [fetus] is healthier."

63. Cf. Pseudo-Galen, *In Hippocratis De alimento commentarius* 4.18 (ed. Kühn, 15:405).

64. Galen, *In Hippocratis Epidemiarum librum 2 commentaria* 6 (CMG 5.10.1; ed. Wenkebach and trans. Pfaff, 408, lines 1ff.; Latin in Deller, trans., "Exzerpta aus Epidemienkommentaren," 528, no. 41). See also Maimonides, *Commentary on Hippocrates' Aphorisms* 5.40 (ed. and trans. Bos, forthcoming): "Says Hippocrates: When blood congeals in the breasts of a woman, it indicates that her condition is [one of] madness."

The Seventeenth Treatise

1. "That is, people do not fall ill . . . move after eating": Cf. Maimonides, *Regimen of Health* 2 (ed. and trans. Bos, forthcoming): "Similarly, Galen has said and these are his very words: If someone wishes not to fall ill at all, he should endeavor not to suffer from indigestion and not to move after a meal."

2. Galen, *De bonis malisque sucis* 3.3–4 (ed. Helmreich, 397, lines 15–20). Aphorisms 17.1–7 are quoted by the seventeenth-century Jewish physician Jacob Zahalon in his commentary to Maimonides' *Hilkhot De°ot*, ch. 4, in the Hebrew translation that he himself prepared from a Latin one; see Zahalon, *Shemirat ha-beri°ut leha-Rambam*, 26–29.

3. Cf. Hippocrates, *Epidemics* 6.4 (ed. and trans. Smith, 239, no. 18): "Healthy discipline, not gluttonizing, not avoiding work." Cf. Maimonides, *Regimen of Health* 1.1 (ed. and trans. Bos, forthcoming): "Note how Hippocrates summarized the entire regimen of health in two rules, namely that a person should not eat until he is satisfied and that he should not neglect exercise."

4. Galen, *In Hippocratis Epidemiarum librum* 6 *commentaria* 1 (CMG 5.10.2.2; ed. Wenkebach and trans. Pfaff, 27, lines 23–24; Latin in Deller, trans., "Exzerpta aus Epidemienkommentaren," 532, no. 59).

5. "because of gluttony": Lit. "because his condition [is one] of gluttony."

6. Galen, *De bonis malisque sucis* 4.39 (ed. Helmreich, 407, lines 4–6).

7. This Pseudo-Galenic treatise survives only in an Arabic translation edited and translated by Nabielek. See Strohmaier, "Der syrische und der arabische Galen," 2015n13. For this quotation, see Pseudo-Galen, *Über Schlaf und Wachsein* (ed. and trans. Nabielek, 34). Also see the introduction to this volume.

8. "so that it provides . . . its temperament": This passage does not appear in Galen, *De sanitate tuenda* 1.3 (ed. Koch, 6, line 20). See the introduction to this volume.

9. Galen, *De sanitate tuenda* 1.3 (ed. Koch, 6, lines 19–22).

10. Galen, *De sanitate tuenda* 1.8 (ed. Koch, 20, lines 1–4).

11. Galen, *In Hippocratis Epidemiarum librum* 6 *commentaria* 6 (CMG 5.10.2.2; ed. Wenkebach and trans. Pfaff, 330, lines 35–37, 17–21; Latin in Deller, trans., "Exzerpta aus Epidemienkommentaren," 543, no. 113).

12. Cf. Galen, *De arte parva* 24 (ed. Kühn, 1:371), and the translation by Boudon-Millot, *Art médical*, 351n9: "According to Epicurus sexual intercourse is not useful for one's health, but in reality there should be such intervals that one does not feel feebleness but that one feels a little lighter and breathes more easily."

13. Galen, *De arte parva* 24 (ed. Kühn, 1:371–72; ed. and trans. Boudon-Millot, 351–52, no. 9). This text originally hails, as Boudon-Millot (p. 351n2) remarks, from a little lost treatise by Galen on aphrodisiacs that is preserved in Oribasius, *Collectiones medicae* 6.37 (see ed. Raeder, 1:187, lines 28–188), and partially in Galen, *De venereis* (see ed. Kühn, 5:911). Boudon-Millot does not deal with Maimonides' quotations in her admirable edition.

14. Galen, *In Hippocratis Epidemiarum librum* 6 *commentaria* 6 (CMG 5.10.2.2; ed. Wenkebach and trans. Pfaff, 306, lines 8–11; Latin in Deller, trans., "Exzerpta aus Epidemienkommentaren," 538, no. 92).

15. Cf. Galen, *De sanitate tuenda* 2.2 (ed. Koch, 39, lines 17–18); translation by Green in *Galen's "Hygiene,"* 53: "For the care of health, work should come first, and should be followed by food, drink, sleep, and sex relations for those who are to engage in it." See aphorism 17.12 as well.

16. Galen, *De sanitate tuenda* 2.2 (ed. Koch, 39, lines 15–17). Cf. Anastassiou and Irmer, eds., *Testimonien zum Corpus Hippocraticum*, pt. 2, 2:217.

17. "overflows the cardia of the stomach": Cf. Galen, *In Hippocratis De acutorum morborum victu commentarius* 3.55 (ed. Helmreich, 263, line 11): ἐπιπολάζειν. Cf. Ullmann, *Wörterbuch zu griechisch-arabischen Übersetzungen*, 259.

18. Galen, *In Hippocratis De acutorum morborum victu commentarius* 3.55 (ed. Helmreich, 263, lines 8–11).

19. This aphorism is possibly an adaptation and partly a repetition of the same Galenic text quoted in aphorism 17.10 above, namely *De sanitate tuenda* 2.2 (ed. Koch, 39, lines 15–16).

20. Galen, *De sanitate tuenda* 6.4 (ed. Koch, p. 176, line 36–p. 177, line 4).

21. This text from Galen's *De sanitate tuenda* 6.14 (ed. Koch, 194, lines 26–36), is quoted by Maimonides with some variations in *On Asthma* 10.8 (ed. and trans. Bos, 55).

22. "he": I.e., someone suffering from a bad constitution.

23. "solid bread": Cf. Galen, *De sanitate tuenda* 6.14 (ed. Koch, 196, line 23): ἄρτον ἄζυμον κριβανιτήν (unleavened bread baked in a pan).

24. Galen, *De sanitate tuenda* 6.14 (ed. Koch, 194, lines 26–36; 196, lines 17–24).

25. Galen, *De alimentorum facultatibus* 2.6.4 (ed. Helmreich, 273, lines 5–8).

26. "One acts prudently and securely": Cf. Galen, *De alimentorum facultatibus* 2.8.5 (ed. Helmreich, 275, line 7): ἀσφαλέστατον.

27. Galen, *De alimentorum facultatibus* 2.8.5 (ed. Helmreich, 275, lines 6–7).

28. Galen, *De sanitate tuenda* 1.7 (ed. Koch, 16, lines 1–5).

29. "sounds": Galen, *De sanitate tuenda* 1.8 (ed. Koch, 19, line 26) adds "and music in general." For this quotation, cf. Maimonides, *On Asthma* 1.2 (ed. and trans. Bos, 6).

30. "Bad humors often cause diseases": Added by Maimonides; not in Galen, *De sanitate tuenda* 1.8.

31. Galen, *De sanitate tuenda* 1.8 (ed. Koch, 19, lines 24–26).

32. Galen, *De sanitate tuenda* 6.7 (ed. Koch, 180, lines 24–25); Galen speaks about the eating habits of those whose constitutions are faultless.

33. This quotation does not feature in Galen, *De sanitate tuenda* 6.7 (ed. Koch, 180, lines 24–25). Following his discussion of the eating habits of those with a perfect constitution, Galen describes the regimen of those whose abdomen is bilious and states that they should have purging foods first and then astringent ones.

34. "educated": Cf. Galen, *De sanitate tuenda* 6.14 (ed. Koch, 197, line 14): τοῖς πεπαιδευμένοις.

35. "activities": Lit. "movements."

36. Galen, *De sanitate tuenda* 6.14 (ed. Koch, 197, lines 2–7, 14–17).

37. This quotation has not been preserved in the spurious text edited by Kühn (Pseudo-Galen, *In Hippocratis De alimento commentarius* 1 [ed. Kühn, 15:224–28]).

38. "Well-prepared": Cf. Galen, *De bonis malisque sucis* 7.1 (ed. Helmreich, 413, line 13): καλῶς ἐσκευασμένη.

39. Galen, *De bonis malisque sucis* 7.1 (ed. Helmreich, 413, lines 12–14).

40. Galen, *De consuetudinibus* (ed. Schmutte, 6; German translation from the Arabic by Pfaff, 41). See also Klein-Franke's edition and translation, p. 129 (English) and p. 141 (Arabic).

41. Galen, *De consuetudinibus* (ed. Schmutte, 16; German translation from the Arabic by Pfaff, 45). See also Klein-Franke's edition and translation, p. 133 (English) and p. 144 (Arabic).

42. See the introduction to this volume.

43. Galen, *De victu attenuante* 12 (ed. Kalbfleisch, 450, lines 16–17).

44. Galen, *De alimentorum facultatibus* 3.27.2 (ed. Helmreich, 367, lines 1–4).

45. Galen, *De sanitate tuenda* 1.11 (ed. Koch, 25, line 31–26, line 4).

46. Galen, *De sanitate tuenda* 1.11 (ed. Koch, 26, lines 4–7).

47. Galen, *De sanitate tuenda* 5.3 (ed. Koch, 141, lines 8–10; 142, lines 6–9).

48. Galen, *De sanitate tuenda* 5.5 (ed. Koch, 144, lines 13–14; 145, lines 1–3). See the introduction to this volume and Anastassiou and Irmer, eds., *Testimonien zum Corpus Hippocraticum*, pt. 2, 2:366.

49. Galen, *De sanitate tuenda* 5.4 (ed. Koch, 143, lines 16–17). The same text is quoted by Maimonides in his *On Asthma* 6.2 (ed. and trans. Bos, 29) and commented upon at length by Maimonides. See also aphorism 20.8 below and Maimonides' *Abridgement of Galen's De sanitate tuenda*, MS Paris 1203, fol. 27b: "When his strength is weak, the body should be fed small amounts at short intervals."

50. This last part of the quotation does not occur in *De sanitate tuenda* 5, but it is found in Maimonides, *On Asthma* 6.2 (ed. and trans. Bos, 29).

51. "perfectly baked": Cf. Galen, *De sanitate tuenda* 5.7 (ed. Koch, 148, line 11): ὠπτημένος τε ἀκριβῶς εἴη.

52. "flatulence develops in the hypochondria": Galen, *De sanitate tuenda* 5.7 (ed. Koch, 150, lines 11–12), speaks about "symptoms in the right hypochondria."

53. Galen, *De sanitate tuenda* 5.7 (ed. Koch, 148, lines 10–11; 150, lines 9–12).

54. Galen, *De sanitate tuenda* 5.8 (ed. Koch, 152, lines 17–18).

55. Galen, *De sanitate tuenda* 5.9 (ed. Koch, 152, line 32). The advice to give them dried figs in winter, as it appears in Galen, is actually part of the text quoted by Maimonides in aphorism 17.32, where Galen recommends dried figs and Damascene plums as additional means to soften the stool in winter, either boiled or simply soaked in honey wine that has added honey, or even better Attic honey.

56. Galen, *De sanitate tuenda* 5.8 (ed. Koch, 152, lines 17–19).

57. Galen, *De sanitate tuenda* 5.9 (ed. Koch, 152, lines 24–28).

58. Galen, *De sanitate tuenda* 5.9 (ed. Koch, 154, lines 8–9). Galen stipulates that it should be given only to those who are constipated during chronic diseases and those similarly constipated during convalescence after long illness.

59. Galen, *De sanitate tuenda* 5.9 (ed. Koch, 152, lines 28–29).

60. Galen, *De sanitate tuenda* 5.9 (ed. Koch, p. 152, line 32–p. 153, line 2). Galen recommends: "Damascene plums, either boiled or simply soaked in honey wine that has added honey, or even better Attic honey" (see n. 55 above).

61. Galen, *De sanitate tuenda* 6.7 (ed. Koch, p. 180, line 32–p. 181, line 4). Galen makes this recommendation to those who have a bilious abdomen.

62. Pseudo-Galen, *In Hippocratis De alimento commentarius* 4.19 (ed. Kühn, 15:406). Cf. aphorism 16.32 above.

63. "that in which old age has just begun": Cf. Galen, *De sanitate tuenda* 5.12 (ed. Koch, 167, lines 18–19): ὃ [τὸ] τῶν ὠμογερόντων (that of active old men).

64. "The second stage . . . mentioned [before]": Cf. Galen, *De sanitate tuenda* 5.12 (ed. Koch, 167, lines 20–23): "and the second portion in which they are called decrepit (σύμφορον τὸ ὄνομα φέρουσι) is that of which they say: When he has bathed and eaten, let him sleep softly."

65. "senility": Cf. Galen, *De sanitate tuenda* 5.12 (ed. Koch, 167, line 28): πέμπελον.

66. "and in which sharp biting [superfluities] . . . in his body": Galen, *De sanitate tuenda* 5.12 (ed. Koch, 167, line 27) adds: "because of their cold constitution."

67. Galen, *De sanitate tuenda* 5.12 (ed. Koch, 167, lines 18–28).

68. Galen, *De marcore* 5 (ed. Kühn, 7:682).

69. "incision": Galen, *De consuetudinibus* (ed. Schmutte, 32, lines 8–9), adds: "in the veins near the ankles or the nose."

70. Galen, *De consuetudinibus* (ed. Schmutte, 32, lines 5–10; German translation by Pfaff from the Arabic, p. 51). See also Klein-Franke's edition and translation, p. 137 (English) and pp. 149–50 (Arabic).

71. Galen, *De consuetudinibus* (ed. Schmutte, 32, lines 12–16; German translation by Pfaff from the Arabic, p. 51). See also Klein-Franke's edition and translation, p. 137 (English) and p. 150 (Arabic).

72. Galen, *De consuetudinibus* (ed. Schmutte, 34, lines 11–14; German translation by Pfaff from the Arabic, p. 52). See also Klein-Franke's edition and translation, p. 138 (English) and p. 150 (Arabic).

73. "*hiera*": Cf. aphorism 16.2 above.

74. "lesser bindweed . . . dried figs and safflower": Galen, *De sanitate tuenda* 5.9 (ed. Koch, 153, lines 18–19), recommends a mercurial herb (λινόζωστις), the so-called sea kale (θαλασσοκράμβη), safflower in barley gruel, and other moderately medicinal drugs.

75. One hazelnut varies from 3.31 to 4.25 grams.

76. Galen, *De sanitate tuenda* 5.9 (ed. Koch, 153, lines 18–26).

77. "If someone complains of constant headache": Galen, *De sanitate tuenda* 6.10 (ed. Koch, 186, line 25), speaks of "those who are in continuous pain" (τὰς μέντοι συνεχῶς). Later on Galen specifies these pains as headaches, symptoms of effusions [of bile into the stomach] and epileptic convulsions (ed. Koch, 187, lines 2–3).

78. "*picra* remedy": A compound drug with aloe as a main component. See Galen, *De sanitate tuenda* 6.10 (ed. Koch, 187, lines 8–9): "the aloe remedy which is called *picra* (i.e., bitter)"; also see aphorism 16.2 above.

79. "nard" (*nārdīn*): Its most important species are Indian valerian (*Nardostachys jatamansi*), Celtic spikenard (*Valeriana celtica*), and wild nard (*Asarum europaeum*; also called asarabacca).

80. Galen, *De sanitate tuenda* 6.10 (ed. Koch, p. 186, line 25–p. 187, line 16).

81. "the cumin stomachic": See Galen, *De sanitate tuenda* 6.7 (ed. Koch, 182, lines 6–7): τό τε Διοσπολιτικὸν ὀνομαζόμενον φάρμακον. Galen adds that niter should be mixed equally with the other ingredients.

82. Galen, *De sanitate tuenda* 6.7 (ed. Koch, 182, lines 3–10).

83. "theriac": A confection originally given as an antidote to snakebite and, later, occasionally as a general tonic. In Galen's *De theriaca ad Pisonem* and Pseudo-Galen's *De theriaca ad Pamphilianum* (ed. Kühn, 14:1–310), we find detailed descriptions of the different theriacs.

84. "an Egyptian bean": I.e., 2.34 grams.

85. Galen, *De theriaca ad Pisonem* 17 (ed. Kühn, 14:285–86; see also ed. and trans. Richter-Bernburg, 96–98 [Arabic], 107–9 [German]). Cf. Anastassiou and Irmer, eds., *Testimonien zum Corpus Hippocraticum*, pt. 2, 2:89 (Hippocrates, *Aphorismes* 4.5 [ed. and trans. Littré, 4:502, line 14 (Greek), 503 (French)]): "Ad Pisonem." The Arabic title *Ilā Qayṣar* is a corruption of *Ilā Fīṣun*. See also Steinschneider, "Griechische Ärzte," 292n55; and Ullmann, *Medizin im Islam*, 49, no. 51.

The Eighteenth Treatise

1. "he does not have to be very careful [about his diet]": Cf. Galen, *De bonis malisque sucis* 2.2 (ed. Helmreich, 394, lines 1–2): οὐδὲ τῆς ἀκριβοῦς πάνυ διαίτης ἐδέησε.

2. Galen, *De bonis malisque sucis* 2.2 (ed. Helmreich, 394, lines 1–4).

3. "And many . . . inflicted on their soul": The sentence seems to be a faulty translation of Galen, *De parvae pilae exercitio* 1 (ed. Kühn, 5:900): πολλοὶ δ' ἑάλωσαν ἀνιαθέτες (but many [others] have fallen ill from grief).

4. Galen, *De parvae pilae exercitio* 1 (ed. Kühn, 5:899–900). Cf. Bos, "Preservation of Health," 221–22.

5. "from hand to hand": I.e., to each other.

6. Galen, *De parvae pilae exercitio* 1 (ed. Kühn, 5:900).

7. Galen, *De parvae pilae exercitio* 1 (ed. Kühn, 5:901–2).

8. "that": I.e., the superfluous material.

9. Galen, *In Hippocratis Aphorismos commentarius* 3.15 (ed. Kühn, 17B:600).

10. Galen, *In Hippocratis Epidemiarum librum 3 commentaria* 3 (ed. Wenkebach and trans. Pfaff, 140, lines 6–9; Latin in Deller, trans., "Exzerpte aus Epidemienkommentaren," 530, no. 50.)

11. Galen, *De sanitate tuenda* 3.12 (ed. Koch, 99, line 22).

12. Galen, *In Hippocratis Aphorismos commentarius* 3.20 (ed. Kühn, 17B:617–18).

13. Galen, *In Hippocratis De natura hominis commentaria tria* 2.1 (ed. Mewaldt, 58, lines 1–2, 29–31).

14. Pseudo-Galen, "Über Schlaf und Wachsein" (ed. and trans. Nabielek, 35). Also see aphorism 17.4 above.

15. "good": Cf. Galen, *De sanitate tuenda* 6.3 (ed. Koch, 172, line 29): μαλακαῖς (gentle).

16. Galen, *De sanitate tuenda* 6.3 (ed. Koch, 172, lines 27–29, 31).

17. Galen, *De sanitate tuenda* 5.3 (ed. Koch, 141, lines 16–18, 20–21). Cf. Anastassiou and Irmer, eds., *Testimonien zum Corpus Hippocraticum*, pt. 2, 2:217 (Hippocrates, *Aphorismes* 5.38 [ed. and trans. Littré, 4:544, lines 11–13 (Greek), 545 (French)]).

18. Galen, *De sanitate tuenda* 2.2 (ed. Koch, 39, lines 30–34). Cf. Maimonides, *On the Regimen of Health* 1.7 (ed. Bos, forthcoming): "Not every movement is exercise, according to the physicians. What they call exercise is a strong or fast movement or a combination of both, that is, a vigorous movement whereby breathing changes and a person begins to breathe heavily." Cf. Bos, "Preservation of Health," 221.

19. Galen, *De sanitate tuenda* 2.2 (ed. Koch, 41, lines 6–9, 17–20).

20. "and you find him moving quickly, while his movements are even": Cf. Galen, *De sanitate tuenda* 2.2 (ed. Koch, 70, lines 31–32): καὶ αἱ κινήσεις ἕτοιμοί τε καὶ ὁμαλαὶ καὶ εὔρυθμοι γίνωνται.

21. Galen, *De sanitate tuenda* 2.2 (ed. Koch, p. 70, line 28–p. 71, line 2).

22. "restorative": Alternatively, "apotherapeutic."

23. The quotation seems to be a selection and adaptation of material taken from Galen, *De sanitate tuenda* 3.3, 4.

24. Galen, *Ad Glauconem de methodo medendi* 12 (ed. Kühn, 11:39).

The Nineteenth Treatise

1. The following section on bathing is quoted in Giunta, ed., *De balneis*.

2. The term *ḥammām* (lit. "bathhouse") can refer to all the activities carried out in it. Cf. Galen, *In Hippocratis Aphorismos commentarius* 3.15 (ed. Kühn, 17B:600): βαλανεῖα.

3. Cf. Galen, *In Hippocratis Aphorismos commentarius* 3.15 (ed. Kühn, 17B:600).

4. "the other types of dryness": I.e., in addition to the consumptive or marasmus-like fever mentioned by Galen previously in *De marcore* 7 (ed. Kühn, 7:695).

5. Galen, *De marcore* 7 (ed. Kühn, 7:695–96).

6. "and one is very hungry": Lit. "and there is a strong need for food."

7. Galen, *De marcore* 9 (ed. Kühn, 7:702–3).

8. Galen, *Ad Glauconem de methodo medendi* 1.15 (ed. Kühn, 11:52–53).

9. The enumeration follows the Hebrew translation by Muntner and the English one by Rosner. According to Muntner, the missing aphorism appears in one of the Arabic manuscripts and deals with bathing once the fever is over.

10. Galen, *De causis morborum liber* 4–5 (ed. Kühn, 7:19–20). Galen's *De morborum causis et symptomatibus* consists of six books: *De morborum differentiis, De causis morborum liber, De symptomatum differentiis liber,* and *De symptomatum causis* 1–3 (cf. Ullmann, *Medizin im Islam*, 42, no. 22).

11. "drinkable": I.e., neither too sweet nor too salty.

12. "of a moderate temperature": I.e., neither too cold nor too hot.

13. Galen, *De sanitate tuenda* 3.4 (ed. Koch, 83, lines 2–7).

14. Galen, *De sanitate tuenda* 3.4 (ed. Koch, 83, lines 15–20).

15. Galen, *In Hippocratis Epidemiarum librum* 6 *commentaria* 5 (CMG 5.10.2.2; ed. Wenkebach and trans. Pfaff, 319, lines 20–22, 25; cf. 320, lines 23–24; Latin translation in Deller, trans., "Exzerpta aus Epidemienkommentaren," 540, no. 96). Cf. Anastassiou and Irmer, eds., *Testimonien zum Corpus Hippocraticum*, pt. 2, 1:258 (Hippocrates, *Sixième livre des épidémies* 4.13 [ed. and trans. Littré, 5:310, line 8 (Greek text), 311 (French translation)]).

16. Galen, *De sanitate tuenda* 4.4 (ed. Koch, 114, lines 8–10).

17. "firmness of the skin" (*istiḥṣāf*): Cf. Galen, *De methodo medendi* 8.2 (ed. Kühn, 10:535): στεγνώσις; translation by Johnston and Horsley, *Method of Medicine*, 2:352–53: "stoppage of the pores."

18. Galen, *De methodo medendi* 8.2 (ed. Kühn, 10:535; Johnston and Horsley, 2:352–55).

19. Galen, *De methodo medendi* 12.3 (ed. Kühn, 10:828–29; ed. and trans. Johnston and Horsley, 3:252–55).

20. Galen, *De methodo medendi* 14.16 (ed. Kühn, 10:999–1000; ed. and trans. Johnston and Horsley, 3:504–7).

21. Galen, *De compositione medicamentorum secundum locos* 2.1 (ed. Kühn, 12:535–36). Galen actually speaks about the cure for headache caused by biting humors accumulating at the cardia of the stomach. For the Arabic *mayāmir*, coined after the Syriac *mēmra*, see Ullmann, *Medizin im Islam*, 48, no. 50.

22. "Those who [professionally] use a high voice": Cf. Galen, *De compositione medicamentorum secundum locos* 7.1 (ed. Kühn, 13:6): οἱ φωνασκοῦντες (singers).

23. Galen, *De compositione medicamentorum secundum locos* 7.1 (ed. Kühn, 13:6–7).

24. Galen, *De methodo medendi* 13.22 (ed. Kühn, 10:937–38; ed. and trans. Johnston and Horsley, 3:412–15).

25. "let him go into the bathing basin": Cf. Galen, *De compositione medicamentorum secundum locos* 9.2 (ed. Kühn, 13:252): "let him take a bath and remain in it for a long time, but his feet should stay outside."

26. Galen, *De compositione medicamentorum secundum locos* 9.2 (ed. Kühn, 13:252).

27. "who cannot enter . . . beginning of the day": The reason he cannot go to the bathhouse immediately after exercise early in the morning, is—as Galen remarks in *De sanitate tuenda* 6.7 (ed. Kühn, 6:411)—that he has a busy life.

28. Galen, *De sanitate tuenda* 6.7 (ed. Kühn, 6:411–12).

29. "omphacine oil": Oil extracted from green, unripe olives.

30. Galen, *De sanitate tuenda* 6.9 (ed. Kühn, 6:411).

31. Galen, *De sanitate tuenda* 6.4 (ed. Kühn, 6:402).

32. Galen, *De sanitate tuenda* 5.12 (ed. Kühn, 6:373).

33. Galen, *De sanitate tuenda* 4.5 (ed. Kühn, 6:263).

34. Galen, *Ad Glauconem de methodo medendi* 1.12 (ed. Kühn, 11:39).

35. Galen, *In Hippocratis Aphorismos commentarius* 7.46 (ed. Kühn, 18A:152).

36. Galen, *In Hippocratis De acutorum morborum victu commentarius* 3.57 (ed. Helmreich, 263, lines 19–22; 264, lines 1–13). Hippocrates remarks that on the whole, bathing benefits pneumonia rather than ardent fevers because it soothes pain in the sides, chest, and back. Galen comments that it is beneficial in the case of some people suffering from ardent fever.

37. Cf. Galen, *De marcore* 7 (ed. Kühn, 7:691) and *De methodo medendi* 8.3 (ed. Kühn, 10:554).

38. This quotation could not be retrieved in this form. Galen remarks that bathing indeed stops diarrhea but at the same time is harmful because it draws superfluous material back into the body. Galen, *In Hippocratis De acutorum morborum victu commentarius* 3.58 (ed. Helmreich, 265, lines 1–2).

39. Galen states that everybody knows that it is better for those who suffer from constipation to excrete the old excrement, just as bathing further reduces the strength of those already weak. Galen, *In Hippocratis De acutorum morborum victu commentarius* 3.58 (ed. Helmreich, 265, lines 2–5).

40. Galen, *In Hippocratis De acutorum morborum victu commentarius* 3.58 (ed. Helmreich, 265, lines 6–8, 10–11).

41. Galen, *In Hippocratis De acutorum morborum victu commentarius* 3.61 (ed. Helmreich, 267, lines 26–28; 268, lines 1–6).

42. Galen, *In Hippocratis De acutorum morborum victu commentarius* 3.52 (ed. Helmreich, 262, lines 14–21). Cf. Anastassiou and Irmer, eds., *Testimonien zum Corpus Hippocraticum*, pt. 2, 1:19 (Hippocrates, *Du Régime dans les Maladies aigues* [ed. and trans. Littré, 2:366, lines 7–8 (Greek text), 367 (French translation)]).

43. Galen, *De marcore* 7 (ed. Kühn, 7:691).

44. Galen, *Ad Glauconem de methodo medendi* 1.3 (ed. Kühn, 11:14).

45. Galen, *Ad Glauconem de methodo medendi* 1.10 (ed. Kühn, 11:32–33).

46. "so that it encourages . . . pleasure to enjoy": The idea seems to be that the nature of the patient—his healing force—is activated and spreads through all the parts of the body because of its attraction to the pleasant water all around the body. Cf. Galen, *De methodo medendi* 7.6 (ed. Kühn, 10:473–74); translation by Johnston and Horsley, 2:262–63: "What is most pleasant calls upon Nature to open out and extend in every direction toward what is pleasant."

47. Galen, *De methodo medendi* 7.6 (ed. Kühn, 10:472–73; ed. and trans. Johnston and Horsley, 2:260–263).

48. Galen, *De methodo medendi* 7.6 (ed. Kühn, 10:479; ed. and trans. Johnston and Horsley, 2:270–71).

49. "because he has been burned by the sun": Cf. Galen, *De methodo medendi* 8.3 (ed. Kühn, 10:554): ἐπ'ἐγκαύσει, and the translation by Johnston and Horsley, 2:282–83: "due to a heat-stroke."

50. Galen, *De methodo medendi* 8.3 (ed. Kühn, 10:554; ed. and trans. Johnston and Horsley, 2:382–83).

51. Galen, *De methodo medendi* 10.10 (ed. Kühn, 10:721–22; ed. and trans. Johnston and Horsley, 3:92–93).

52. Galen, *De methodo medendi* 11.9 (ed. Kühn, 10:760; ed. and trans. Johnston and Horsley, 3:150–51).

53. Galen, *De methodo medendi* 11.20 (ed. Kühn, 10:803; ed. and trans. Johnston and Horsley, 3:212–13).

54. Galen, *De methodo medendi* 11.20–21 (ed. Kühn, 10:805–6; ed. and trans. Johnston and Horsley, 3:216–19).

55. Galen, *De sanitate tuenda* 6.3 (ed. Koch, 172, lines 20–34).

56. Galen, *De sanitate tuenda* 6.3 (ed. Koch, p. 172, line 33–p. 173, line 4).

The Twentieth Treatise

1. "that the chyme produced . . . all the other organs": Cf. Galen, *De bonis malisque sucis* 10.4 (ed. Helmreich, 419, lines 23–25): "that the chyme produced from the digestion of food fits the temperament of the other organs."

2. Galen, *De bonis malisque sucis* 10.4 (ed. Helmreich, 419, lines 20–25).

3. Galen, *De alimentorum facultatibus* 1.1.1 (ed. Helmreich, p. 201, line 5–p. 202, line 2).

4. Galen, *De alimentorum facultatibus* 1.2.8, 9 (ed. Helmreich, 220, lines 9–10, 18–20).

5. "through its specific substance and nature": Cf. Galen, *De alimentorum facultatibus* 2.6.2 (ed. Helmreich, 272, line 10): τῆς οὐσίας, and translation by Grant in *Food and Diet*, 114: "the uniqueness of their composition."

6. "or through the occurrence of a symptom": Cf. Galen, *De alimentorum facultatibus* 2.6.2 (ed. Helmreich, 272, line 10): ἢ κατά τι σύμπτωμα τῇ πείρᾳ κριτέον, and translation by Grant in *Food and Diet*, 114: "or through some attribute that surfaces during testing."

7. Galen, *De alimentorum facultatibus* 2.6.2 (ed. Helmreich, 272, lines 9–10).

8. Galen, *De alimentorum facultatibus* 2.51.5 (ed. Helmreich, 317, lines 15–21).

9. Galen, *De alimentorum facultatibus* 3.32 (ed. Helmreich, p. 376, line 20–p. 377, line 5), remarks that while the meat of oysters is the softest of the testaceans and relaxes the stomach more, it is less nourishing. Testaceans with hard meat, he says, are more difficult to digest and to dissolve but are more nourishing.

10. Galen, *De alimentorum facultatibus* 2.51.5 (ed. Helmreich, 317, lines 15–21). Also see the introduction to this volume.

11. "with continuous fever": See Galen, *De propriorum animi cuiuslibet affectuum dignotione et curatione* (ed. Boer, 21, line 14): πυρετῷ συνεχεῖ. **BELOU** read "with fever all of a sudden."

12. Galen, *De propriorum animi cuiuslibet affectuum dignotione et curatione* (ed. Boer, 21, lines 12–19).

13. Galen, *De methodo medendi* 7.6 (ed. Kühn, 10:489–91; ed. and trans. Johnston and Horsley, 2:284–87).

14. "day": Lit. "night."

15. Galen, *De methodo medendi* 7.6 (ed. Kühn, 10:489–90; ed. and trans. Johnston and Horsley, 2:284–87).

16. Cf. **C**: "For he [Hippocrates] would not have a grain of common sense if he did not know that putrid foods and beverages produce corruption similar to that produced by fatal poisons." Galen's commentary on this Hippocratic treatise survives only in an Arabic translation (ed. Strohmaier, forthcoming); our quotation does not appear in the Hebrew translation by Solomon ha-Meʾati (ed. Wasserstein). I thank Professor Strohmaier for providing me with photocopies of the passages from his forthcoming edition.

17. This quotation has not been preserved in the spurious text Pseudo-Galen, *In Hippocratis De alimento commentarius* 2 (ed. Kühn, 15:229–50). See aphorism 16.32 above.

18. "weakness of the body . . . temperament of the body": Missing in Kühn's spurious edition of Pseudo-Galen, *In Hippocratis De alimento commentarius* 4.25 (ed. Kühn, 15:412). Cf. aphorism 16.32 above.

19. Pseudo-Galen, *In Hippocratis De alimento commentarius* 4.25 (ed. Kühn, 15:412).

20. On the laxative power of scammony, cf. Maimonides, *Treatise on Logic* 8 (ed. and trans. Efros, 40, lines 16–17 [Hebrew], 48 [English]): "In like manner, all the results of experience, e.g., that scammony is a cathartic and gall-nut causes constipation, are also true."

21. "have": Lit. "are composed and combined of." Cf. Galen, *De alimentorum facultatibus* 1.1.25 (ed. Helmreich, 209, line 16): μικτὴ.

22. "any of these influences": I.e., heating, cooling, drying, and moistening. See Galen, *De alimentorum facultatibus* 1.1.25 (ed. Helmreich, 209, line 25).

23. "but those that exist are merely nourishing": Galen, *De alimentorum facultatibus* 1.1.25 (ed. Helmreich, 210, lines 2–4) adds "since they do not change the body in quality when ingested."

24. Galen, *De alimentorum facultatibus* 1.1.25 (ed. Helmreich, p. 209, lines 12–17, 21–23, 25–p. 210, line 3). Cf. Anastassiou and Irmer, eds., *Testimonien zum Corpus Hippocraticum*, pt. 2, 2:39 (Hippocrates, *De l'Aliment* 19 [ed. and trans. Littré, 9:104, line 11 (Greek), 105 (French)]).

25. "This is the main thing" (*wa-hādhā malāk al-amr*): Cf. Galen, *De alimentorum facultatibus* 2.6.3 (ed. Helmreich, 272, line 24): ἔστι δ' ἐν τούτῳ μάλιστα τὸ χρήσιμον. See also Maimonides, *On Asthma* 5.1 (ed. and trans. Bos, 24).

26. Galen, *De alimentorum facultatibus* 2.6.3–4 (ed. Helmreich, p. 272, line 21–p. 273, line 5).

27. "oven": Lit. "fire."

28. "pure bread": I.e., white bread made from fine flour, without bran. See aphorism 20.62 below.

29. Galen, *De alimentorum facultatibus* 1.2.3 (ed. Helmreich, 218, lines 4–6).

30. "for someone who does not engage in physical exercise": Cf. Galen, *De alimentorum facultatibus* 1.2.7 (ed. Helmreich, 219, line 28): ἰδιώτῃ.

31. "baked": Lit. "cooked."

32. "But completely unleavened bread is not appropriate for anyone": Cf. Maimonides, *On Asthma* 3.2 (ed. and trans. Bos, 13).

33. Galen, *De alimentorum facultatibus* 1.2.7 (ed. Helmreich, p. 219, line 28–p. 220, line 1).

34. "washed bread": I.e., a light form of bread. Cf. Galen, *De alimentorum facultatibus* 1.8.2 (ed. Helmreich, 228, line 11): πλυτός ἄρτος. See Galen, *De alimentorum facultatibus* 1.5 for a discussion of its properties.

35. "inasmuch as it provides only a little nourishment to the body": According to Galen, *De alimentorum facultatibus* 1.8.2 (ed. Helmreich, 228, line 12), starch provides less nourishment to the body than washed bread.

36. Galen, *De alimentorum facultatibus* 1.8.2 (ed. Helmreich, 228, lines 11–13).

37. Galen, *De naturalibus facultatibus* 1.10 (ed. Brock, 36–37).

38. Galen, *De bonis malisque sucis* 6.8–9 (ed. Helmreich, p. 412, line 27–p. 413, line 2). Cf. Levinger, "Maimonides' *Guide* on Forbidden Food," 198; Lieber,

"Maimonides, the Medical Humanist," 58; and Maimonides, *Medical Aphorisms* 25.10 (ed. and trans. Bos, forthcoming).

39. Galen, *In Hippocratis Epidemiarum librum* 6 *commentaria* 6 (CMG 5.10.2.2; ed. Wenkebach and trans. Pfaff, 356, lines 38–40; 357, lines 11–12; Latin in Deller, trans., "Exzerpta aus Epidemienkommentaren," 541, no. 103). Cf. Anastassiou and Irmer, eds., *Testimonien zum Corpus Hippocraticum*, pt. 2, 1:268 (Hippocrates, *Sixième Livre des Épidémies* 6.5 [ed. and trans. Littré, 5:324, line 13 (Greek), 325 (French)]).

40. This quotation could not be retrieved from the spurious text Pseudo-Galen, *In Hippocratis De alimento commentarius* 4 (ed. Kühn, 15:375–417). Cf. aphorisms 20.11–12 above.

41. Galen, *De alimentorum facultatibus* 3.1.16 (ed. Helmreich, 336, lines 12–15).

42. "taste bad and produce bad [humors]": Cf. Galen, *De alimentorum facultatibus* 3.6.2 (ed. Helmreich, 342, lines 1–2): δύσπεπτοι καὶ κακόχυμοι (are difficult to digest and produce bad humors).

43. Galen, *De alimentorum facultatibus* 3.6.2 (ed. Helmreich, 342, lines 1–9).

44. "food": I.e., meat.

45. "live": Lit. "graze."

46. Galen, *De alimentorum facultatibus* 3.13.1–2 (ed. Helmreich, p. 344, line 27–p. 345, line 7).

47. Galen, *In Hippocratis Aphorismos commentarius* 7.56 (ed. Kühn, 18A:169).

48. "twitching in the temples": Cf. Galen, *In Hippocratis De acutorum morborum victu commentarius* 2.34 (ed. Helmreich, 193, line 14): παλμὸν ἰεβῶν, "twitching in the veins," and variant M (p. 193): παλμὸν κροτάφων, "twitching in the temples."

49. Galen, *In Hippocratis De acutorum morborum victu commentarius* 2.34 (ed. Helmreich, 193, lines 12–15).

50. Galen, *In Hippocratis Epidemiarum librum* 2 *commentaria* 6 (CMG 5.10.1; ed. Wenkebach and trans. Pfaff, 404, lines 40–43; Latin in Deller, trans., "Exzerpta aus Epidemienkommentaren," 528 no. 39).

51. Galen, *In Hippocratis Epidemiarum librum* 6 *commentaria* 6 (CMG 5.10.2.2; ed. Wenkebach and trans. Pfaff, 370, lines 25–27, 34–36; Latin in Deller, trans., "Exzerpta aus Epidemienkommentaren," 541 no. 104).

52. Cf. Galen, *De victu attenuante* 12 (ed. Kalbfleisch, 447, lines 17–18): "Thick, black, sweet wines fill the vessels with thick blood."

53. Galen, *De victu attenuante* 12 (ed. Kalbfleisch, 447, lines 17–22).

54. Galen, *De sanitate tuenda* 4.6 (ed. Koch, 121, lines 28–29).

55. Aphorisms 20.30–33 below are found in an additional section at the end of the treatise in **G**. See the introduction to this volume.

56. Galen, *De methodo medendi* 7.6 (ed. Kühn, 10:483–84; ed. and trans. Johnston and Horsley, 2:276–77); cf. Anastassiou and Irmer, eds., *Testimonien zum Corpus Hippocraticum*, pt. 2, 2:23, 363 (Hippocrates, *Du Régime dans les Maladies aigues* [ed. and trans. Littré 2:344, line 8 (Greek), 345 (French)]).

57. Galen, *De compositione medicamentorum secundum locos* 8.7 (ed. Kühn, 13:200–201).

58. Cf. Galen, *In Hippocratis De natura hominis* 3.12 (ed. Mewaldt, 99, lines 5–7): "Nor is [having] a cold drink after gymnastics without having a warm

drink first harmless, for it harms the stomach and liver, and in some people, the nerves." Galen comments upon Hippocrates' advice concerning a slimming diet for fat people—that they should first exercise on an empty stomach, then drink diluted wine that is not very cold, and then eat.

59. Galen, *In Hippocratis De natura hominis* 3.12 (ed. Mewaldt, 99, lines 5–7).

60. Cf. **C**: "Hippocrates says: All waters originating from snow and ice are bad, because once they are frozen they never regain their original nature, because the light, sweet, and pure part of the water has escaped and fled from becoming frozen while the turbid part has stayed in its condition." See also Solomon ha-Meʾati's Hebrew translation of Galen, *Commentary on Airs, Waters, Places* (ed. and trans. Wasserstein, 64–65).

61. Cf. **C**: "He means the water that is similar to snow and ice in coldness, for it is close to these and is thick and hard and slow to digest."

62. "All turbid water . . . because of the cold": Not in **C**.

63. "Rainwater . . . no use whatsoever for it": Cf. **C**: "When this water starts to putrefy and spoil, cooking is of no use whatsoever to it. Something should be done to it to dispel its putrefaction. [. . .] Therefore, it should be mixed and boiled with skimmed honey." See also Solomon ha-Meʾati's Hebrew translation of Galen, *Commentary on Airs, Waters, Places* (ed. and trans. Wasserstein, 62–63).

64. Galen, *In Hippocratis Epidemiarum librum 6 commentaria* 4 (CMG 5.10.2.2; ed. Wenkebach and trans. Pfaff, 210, lines 19ff.; Latin in Deller, trans., "Exzerpta aus Epidemienkommentaren," 536 no. 79).

65. Galen, *De compositione medicamentorum secundum locos* 7.21 (ed. Kühn, 13:45), remarks that some people add boiled poppy heads to the rainwater so that it does not change into another kind of putrefying quality.

66. Galen, *De compositione medicamentorum secundum locos* 7.21 (ed. Kühn, 13:45).

67. "for anyone [whatever his age]": Cf. Galen, *De sanitate tuenda* 1.11 (ed. Koch, 27, lines 8–9): πάσαις ταῖς ἡλικίαις.

68. Galen, *De sanitate tuenda* 1.11 (ed. Koch, 26, lines 26–29; 27, lines 6–9).

69. Galen, *In Hippocratis Epidemiarum librum 2 commentaria* 6 (CMG 5.10.1; ed. Wenkebach and trans. Pfaff, 400, lines 1–4, 38–40; Latin in Deller, trans., "Exzerpta aus Epidemienkommentaren," 528 no. 38).

70. This quotation could not be found in the spurious text of Pseudo-Galen, *In Hippocratis De alimento commentarius* 4 (ed. Kühn, 15:375–417); it does not appear in the sections on milk on pp. 393–95, 399, 401–2, 405. See aphorism 16.32 above.

71. Galen, *De bonis malisque sucis* 4.27 (ed. Helmreich, 404, lines 14–15).

72. Galen, *De bonis malisque sucis* 4.4, 8 (ed. Helmreich, 398, lines 23–27; 399, lines 20–23). Cf. Levinger, "Maimonides' *Guide* on Forbidden Food," 207.

73. "curdled": Lit. "thickened."

74. This text does not appear in Galen's *De bonis malisque sucis*. It bears some resemblance to *De victu attenuante* 12 (ed. Kalbfleisch, 451, lines 5–14); translation by Singer in *Galen: Selected Works*, 323–24: "The thickest sort of milk is that which is most like cheese, such as cows' or pigs' milk, and the thinnest is the most whey-like—for example asses' milk. . . . But if one adds honey, salt, or both, it will be much thinner. It is thus clear that asses' milk taken with salt or honey is the least

thick-humoured, and this will do no harm to the user of the thinning diet. All other sorts of milk, however, should be avoided."

75. Galen, *De alimentorum facultatibus* 3.14.1 (ed. Helmreich, 345, lines 11–14).

76. "for the chest and lungs": Lit. "for the sites of the chest and lungs." Cf. *Galen, De alimentorum facultatibus* 3.14.13 (ed. Helmreich, 348, line 16): τοῖς δὲ κατὰ θώρακα καὶ πνεύμονα χωρίοις. As a medical term, χωρίον can also mean "part of the body" (Liddell and Scott, *Greek-English Lexicon*, 9th ed., 2016); see also Ullmann, *Wörterbuch zu griechisch-arabischen Übersetzungen: Supplement*, 2:718.

77. "for the [parts below the cartilage of the] ribs": Cf. Galen, *De alimentorum facultatibus* 3.14.13 (ed. Helmreich, 348, line 18): τοῖς ὑποχονδρίοις (for the parts below the cartilage and above the navel, abdomen).

78. Galen, *De alimentorum facultatibus* 3.14.13 (ed. Helmreich, 348, lines 16–18).

79. "and does not provide . . . [as all other cheeses do]": Cf. Galen, *De alimentorum facultatibus* 3.16.3 (ed. Helmreich, 354, lines 18–19): οὐ μὴν οὐδὲ κακόχυμός ἐστιν οὐδὲ πάνυ σφόδρα παχύχυμος, ὅπερ ἁπάντων τυρῶν ἐστι κοινὸν ἔγκλημα (It does not make bad juices, nor extremely thick juices, a common defect of all other cheeses).

80. Galen, *De alimentorum facultatibus* 3.16.3 (ed. Helmreich, 354, lines 13–19).

81. Galen, *In Hippocratis Epidemiarum librum 6 commentaria* 5 (CMG 5.10.2.2; ed. Wenkebach and trans. Pfaff, 299, lines 16–20; Latin in Deller, trans., "Exzerpta aus Epidemienkommentaren," 539 no. 91).

82. "Lettuce . . . good and bad": Cf. Galen, *De bonis malisque sucis* 8.9 (ed. Helmreich, 416, lines 13–14): "Lettuce is in the middle between having good and bad chymes."

83. "turnip [*Brassica rapa*]": The Arabic *lift* can also refer to rape [*Brassica napus*]; see also *Wörterbuch der klassischen arabischen Sprache*, 2:970a, line 30.

84. Galen, *De bonis malisque sucis* 8.9 (ed. Helmreich, 416, lines 13–15).

85. Galen, *De bonis malisque sucis* 8.7 (ed. Helmreich, 416, lines 3–6).

86. "vegetables": Lit. "things."

87. "parsley [*Petroselinum* spp.]": For this vegetable, Arabic *maqdūnis* or *baqdūnis*, see Maimonides, *Glossary of Drug Names*, no. 196 (trans. Rosner); and Dioscurides, *Dioscurides triumphans* 3.63 (ed. and trans. Dietrich, 2:414–15, esp. 415n2).

88. "mountain mint [perhaps *Nepeta cataria* and var.]": See Dioscurides, *Dioscurides triumphans* 3.35 (ed. and trans. Dietrich, 2:382–83, esp. 383n3).

89. "oregano" (*saʿtar*): This name designates numerous species of Labiatae of the oregano, thyme, and savory types. See Maimonides, *Glossary of Drug Names*, no. 319 (trans. Rosner); and Dioscurides, *Dioscurides triumphans* 3.29 (ed. and trans. Dietrich, 2:375–76).

90. "lesser calamint [*Clinopodium nepeta* and var.]": Dietrich, in his translation of Dioscurides, *Dioscurides triumphans* 3.36 (pp. 2:383–85), remarks that this is perhaps identical with *Satureja calaminta* or *Thymus serpyllum*; but according to Kahl, ed. and trans., in the *Dispensatory of Ibn al-Tilmīḏ*, 325, 343, it is calamint (*Calamintha sylvatica*).

91. "fresh": Galen, *De victu attenuante* 2 (ed. Kalbfleisch, 434, line 19), adds "rather than dried."

92. "water parsnip (that is, water celery [perhaps *Sium latifolium* . . . and var.])": The identification of this plant is uncertain. Cf. Maimonides, *Glossary of Drug Names*, no. 340 (trans. Rosner) and Dietrich in Dioscurides, *Dioscurides triumphans* 3.61 (ed. and trans. Dietrich, 2:412–14).

93. "seed of mountain celery": Although Arabic *faṭrāsāliyūn* is often considered to be synonymous with *maqdūnis* or *baqdūnis* (see Dioscurides, *Dioscurides triumphans* 3.63 [ed. and trans. Dietrich, 2:414–15]), it seems that Maimonides, in accordance with the physicians of the Maghreb, considers it to be a different species, namely, the seed of mountain celery. This identification concurs with al-Bustānī, *Muḥīṭ al-Muḥīṭ*, 2:1617b: *al-fuṭrāsāliyūn: bizr al-karafs al-jabalī*. I thank Dr. David Calabro for pointing out this possibility.

94. "blackberry [Br. bramble; *Rubus fruticosus*]": Galen, *De victu attenuante* 2 (ed. Kalbfleisch, 434, line 27), reads "beet" (τεῦτλα).

95. Galen, *De victu attenuante* 2 (ed. Kalbfleisch, 434, lines 15–19, 26–27).

96. Galen, *De victu attenuante* 5 (ed. Kalbfleisch, 437, lines 24–29, 31–32).

97. Galen, *De bonis malisque sucis* 8.1–3 (ed. Helmreich, 414, lines 25–28; 415, lines 1–2, 5–6, 16–17).

98. Cf. Galen, *De victu attenuante* 12 (ed. Kalbfleisch, p. 446, line 33–p. 447, line 2).

99. Cf. Galen, *De victu attenuante* 2 (ed. Kalbfleisch, 435, lines 1–4).

100. "If mulberries [*Morus alba* var. *nigra*] do not pass quickly": Cf. Galen, *De alimentorum facultatibus* 2.11.4 (ed. Helmreich, p. 283, line 24–p. 284, line 2); and the translation by Grant in *Food and Diet*, 122: "but eaten second after other foods, or meeting with a bad juice in the stomach."

101. "gourds": For the different species, see Dioscurides, *Dioscurides triumphans* 2.116 (ed. and trans. Dietrich, 2:282); and Maimonides, *Glossary of Drug Names*, no. 332 (trans. Rosner).

102. Galen, *De alimentorum facultatibus* 2.11.4 (ed. Helmreich, p. 283, line 24–p. 284, line 6).

103. "sharpness": Lit. "cutting."

104. Galen, *De alimentorum facultatibus* 2.26.20 (ed. Helmreich, 296, lines 20–23; 297, lines 11–13).

105. "specific property": This term is especially used by Maimonides for those remedies that operate through the whole of their essence, contrary to remedies that operate either through their matter or through their quality. While the pharmacological action of these remedies can be assessed by a physician, this is not the case with the remedies effective through their specific property that lack a pharmacological basis. Thus, their effectiveness can be learned only through experience. In a lengthy theoretical discussion in his *Commentary on Hippocrates' Aphorisms* 1.12, Maimonides calls the specific property through which these remedies are effective their "specific form" (*al-ṣūrah al-nawʿiya*). See also Maimonides, *On Poisons* 15 (ed. and trans. Bos, 16); and *On Hemorrhoids* 2.3 (ed. and trans. Bos, 10). In his *Medical Aphorisms* 22, Maimonides gives a long list of remedies effective through their specific properties, mostly consisting of all sorts of animals and their parts, excrement, and urine. The subject is discussed in Schwartz, "Magiyah, maddaᶜ nisyoni u-metodah maddaᶜit," 35–38; Ibn Ezra,

Sefer Hanisyonot, 17–20; Langermann, "Gersonides on the Magnet," 273–74; and Bos, introduction to Maimonides, *Medical Aphorisms* 22–25 (forthcoming).

106. Galen, *De compositione medicamentorum secundum locos* 2.1 (ed. Kühn, 12:517).

107. Galen, *De alimentorum facultatibus* 2.27.1; 2.28.1, 3 (ed. Helmreich, 297, lines 19–20; 298, lines 8–9, 18–19).

108. "their substance is similar and conformable to the nature of the liver": Cf. Galen, *De compositione medicamentorum secundum locos* 8.7 (ed. Kühn, 13:200): καθ᾽ ὅλην τὴν οὐσίαν οἰκεία τῷ σπλάγχνῳ (They are, according to their whole substance, conformable to the inward parts).

109. "correct": Lit. "balance."

110. Galen, *De compositione medicamentorum secundum locos* 8.7 (ed. Kühn, 13:200).

111. "most similar to blood": Cf. Galen, *De bonis malisque sucis* 3.1 (ed. Helmreich, 396, line 16): Ἀμεμπτότατα (utterly blameless, most perfect).

112. "and gently boiled eggs": Not in Galen, *De bonis malisque sucis* 3.1.

113. Galen, *De bonis malisque sucis* 3.1 (ed. Helmreich, 396, lines 16–18, 20–21; 397, lines 1–3).

114. "gruel from wheat or spelt" (*khandarūs*): The term, a transcription of the Greek χόνδρος (see Galen, *De methodo medendi* 8.2 [ed. Kühn, 10:548; ed. and trans. Johnston and Horsley, 2:372–73]), can also refer to the groats used for the gruel. Cf. Dioscurides, *Dioscurides triumphans* 2.80 (ed. and trans. Dietrich, 2:247).

115. "oven" (*tannūr*): I.e., an oven excavated in the ground in a circular form. See Maimonides, *On Asthma* 3.1 (ed. and trans. Bos, 11); and Galen, *De methodo medendi* 8.2 (ed. Kühn, 10:548; ed. and trans. Johnston and Horsley, 2:372): οἱ κριβανῖται.

116. "those that live among the rocks": Cf. Galen, *De methodo medendi* 8.2 (ed. Kühn, 10:548; ed. and trans. Johnston and Horsley, 2:374): οἱ πετραῖοι.

117. "partridge" (*ṭayhūj*): The common Arabic term for partridge is *ḥajal*. Cf. Galen, *De methodo medendi* 8.2 (ed. Kühn, 10:549; ed. and trans. Johnston and Horsley, 2:374): πέρδικες.

118. Galen, *De methodo medendi* 8.2 (ed. Kühn, 10:546, 548–49; ed. and trans. Johnston and Horsley, 2:372–75).

119. "vigor": Lit. "abundance." Cf. Galen, *De bonis malisque sucis* 3.4 (ed. Helmreich, 397, lines 26–27): εὐεξίας σώματος. Galen contrasts the normal healthy bodily condition of an ordinary person with the abnormal high condition of the body of an athlete.

120. Galen, *De bonis malisque sucis* 2.9; 3.2, 4 (ed. Helmreich, 396, lines 12–15; 397, lines 6–9, 25–27).

121. "[all] types of bread . . . kneaded, or baked": Cf. Maimonides, *On Asthma* 3.1 (ed. and trans. Bos, 11).

122. "also all types of cheese": Cf. Galen, *De bonis malisque sucis* 4.1 (ed. Helmreich, 398, lines 1–5); and Maimonides, *On Asthma* 3.4 (ed. and trans. Bos, 14).

123. Galen, *De bonis malisque sucis* 4.1, 2, 12, 13, 15, 16, 34, 42 (ed. Helmreich, 398, lines 1–5, 7; 400, lines 14–15, 25; 401, lines 19–20; 402, lines 3, 5–6; 405, lines 26–28; 407, lines 25–26).

124. "practices moderation in his lifestyle": Cf. Galen, *De bonis malisque sucis* 13.3 (ed. Helmreich, 427, line 15): σωφροσύνην δ' ἀσκῶν.

125. Galen, *De bonis malisque sucis* 13.1–3 (ed. Helmreich, p. 427, lines 1–13, 15–p. 428, line 5).

126. "pure bread": I.e., bread prepared from pure flour (without bran); see aphorism 20.15 above.

127. Galen, *De alimentorum facultatibus* 1.2.11 (ed. Helmreich, p. 220, line 29–p. 221, line 4).

128. Galen, *De alimentorum facultatibus* 1.23.4 (ed. Helmreich, 250, lines 16–19).

129. "[This is the case] . . . water and the like": Cf. Galen, *De alimentorum facultatibus* 2.62.1–2 (ed. Helmreich, 325, lines 12–15), and the translation by Grant in *Food and Diet*, 149: "It is vital always to remember this advice and to ascertain whether each of the foods being tested loses during boiling or baking or frying its strong qualities."

130. Galen, *De alimentorum facultatibus* 2.62.1–2 (ed. Helmreich, 325, lines 8–15).

131. "such as the [different kinds of] fat": Not in Galen, *De alimentorum facultatibus* 3.26.3 (ed. Helmreich, 365, line 20).

132. Galen, *De alimentorum facultatibus* (ed. Helmreich, 365, lines 20–23).

133. The text seems to be an adaptation of Galen, *De simplicium medicamentorum temperamentis ac facultatibus* 4.10, 15 (ed. Kühn, 11:651, 669–70). See also Maimonides, *On the Regimen of Health* 4.24 (ed. and trans. Bos, forthcoming): "One should endeavor to take sweet foods, for the sweet is what nourishes, as Galen has mentioned."

134. Abū Marwān ᶜAbd al-Malik ibn Zuhr (d. 1162), known in the West as Avenzoar, was one of the foremost physicians of the Western Caliphate. Born in Seville, he spent most of his life there and was in the service of the Almoravid dynasty. See Colin, *Avenzoar: Sa vie et ses oeuvres*, 23–41; Ullmann, *Medizin im Islam*, 162–63; *Encyclopaedia of Islam*, new ed., s.v. "Ibn Zuhr"; and Kuhne, "Abū Marwān b. Zuhr: Un professionel." Ibn Zuhr is frequently quoted by Maimonides, who regarded him highly. In *Elucidation of Some Symptoms* 2, he praises Avenzoar as "unique in his generation and one of the greatest observers." In *On Poisons* 78 (ed. and trans. Bos, 54) Maimonides remarks: "All this was mentioned and verified by the venerable Abū Marwān b. Zuhr, may God have mercy on him, with his lengthy experience, because he was the greatest among men in testing drugs and one who devoted himself to this more than any other. He was able to do so more than any other because of his great wealth and his skill in the medical art." See also Maimonides, "Medizinischer Schwanengesang" (ed. Kroner, 88–89); Maimonides, *On Asthma* 9.1 (ed. and trans. Bos, 40, 131); and Bos, "Maimonides' Medical Works and Their Contribution," 251–52, 259–60.

135. "that have been confirmed by testing": **BEL** reads: "which he had tested," while **OU** reads: "which I tested."

136. "*Book on Foods* which he composed for one of the Almoravid kings": This is Ibn Zuhr's *Kitāb al-aghdhiya*, edited and translated by Expiración García Sánchez in 1992. It was commissioned by the caliph Abū Muḥammad ᶜAbd al-Muᵓmin ibn ᶜAlī (ruled AH 524–58/1130–63 CE). Cf. Ullmann, *Medizin im Islam*, 201.

137. The father of Abū Marwān ibn Zuhr was Abū l-ʿAlāʾ ibn Zuhr (d. 1131). Cf. Colin, *Avenzoar: Sa vie et ses oeuvres,* 16–22; Ullmann, *Medizin im Islam,* 162; and *Encyclopaedia of Islam,* new ed., s.v. "Ibn Zuhr" [Arnaldez]. The *Kitāb al-tadhkira,* supposedly by the father, was edited and translated by Gabriel Colin in 1911 as *La Teḏkira d'Abū al-ʿAlāʾ*; but on the basis of her research into the existing manuscripts of this text, Cristina Álvarez Millán suggests in "Corpus médico-literario de los Banū Zuhr," 174–75, that the author of this text was not the elder ibn Zuhr, but rather his son, Abū Marwān. See also Maimonides, *Medical Aphorisms* 13.44 (ed. and trans. Bos, 3:49), where Maimonides quotes *waṣāyā* ("rules in hortatory form") by Abū l-ʿAlāʾ ibn Zuhr.

138. Cf. Ibn Zuhr, *Kitāb al-aghdhiya* (ed. García Sánchez, 15).

139. "It fattens the body of the emaciated and convalescents": Not in Ibn Zuhr, *Kitāb al-aghdhiya.*

140. "hens": Ibn Zuhr, *Kitāb al-aghdhiya,* 15, adds "especially fat ones."

141. "and roosters": Missing in Ibn Zuhr, *Kitāb al-aghdhiya.*

142. Cf. Ibn Zuhr, *Kitāb al-aghdhiya,* 15–17.

143. "Sparrows": The Arabic term *ʿaṣāfīr* can also have the more general meaning of small birds.

144. "paralysis": Found in Ibn Zuhr, *Kitāb al-aghdhiya,* 16, and in **m**.

145. "and fly around freely": Lit. "and spread their wings to fly." Ibn Zuhr, *Kitāb al-aghdhiya,* 16, reads "seeking shelter in towers."

146. Ibn Zuhr, *Kitāb al-aghdhiya,* 22–23.

147. "gazelles": Cf. Ibn Zuhr, *Kitāb al-aghdhiya,* 22–23: "female gazelles."

148. "resuscitates": Lit. "cures."

149. Cf. Ibn Zuhr, *Kitāb al-aghdhiya,* 133.

150. Ibn Zuhr, *Kitāb al-aghdhiya,* 19.

151. "turnip": See aphorism 20.47 above.

152. Cf. Ibn Zuhr, *Kitāb al-aghdhiya,* 30, 45.

153. Ibn Zuhr, *Kitāb al-aghdhiya,* 45–46.

154. "and in the muscles": Cf. Ibn Zuhr, *Kitāb al-aghdhiya,* 45–46: "and pains in the muscles."

155. Cf. Ibn Zuhr, *Kitāb al-aghdhiya,* 46–47.

156. Cf. Ibn Zuhr, *Kitāb al-aghdhiya,* 48.

157. "if sour pomegranates . . . in the stomach": Cf. Ibn Zuhr, *Kitāb al-aghdhiya,* 48: "If one takes the thickened juice of sour pomegranates, it is good for the corruption of the foods in the stomach."

158. Cf. Ibn Zuhr, *Kitāb al-aghdhiya,* 51–52.

159. "If used for cooking, . . . [without any superfluities]": Cf. Ibn Zuhr, *Kitāb al-aghdhiya,* 51–52: "When it is put into food, it produces a moisture in it that is free of superfluities."

160. Cf. Ibn Zuhr, *Kitāb al-aghdhiya,* 53.

161. Cf. Ibn Zuhr, *Kitāb al-aghdhiya,* 53–54.

162. "and have the special property of producing hemorrhoids": Cf. Ibn Zuhr, *Kitāb al-aghdhiya,* 53–54: "and cause inflammations in the intestines and liver."

163. The text quoted by Maimonides bears no resemblance to the statements about sesame found in Ibn Zuhr, *Kitāb al-aghdhiya,* 13, 98, 112.

164. "fattens": Lit. "enlarges."

165. Cf. Ibn Zuhr, *Kitāb al-aghdhiya*, 57.

166. The physician al-Tamīmī (d. 980), hailing from Jerusalem, moved to Egypt in 970 to serve the vizier Yaʿqūb ibn Killis. His *Kitāb al-murshid fī jawāhir al-aghdhiya wa-quwā l-mufradāt min al-adwiya* (Guide to the substances of foods and the powers of simple drugs) has been only partly preserved and is for the most part still in manuscript form; cf. Ullmann, *Medizin im Islam*, 269–70.

167. See the introduction to this volume.

168. "that are separated from their mother" (*al-muḥtalima*): The Arabic term is normally used for referring to someone reaching puberty.

169. "Soup prepared . . . and for asthma": Cf. Maimonides, *On Asthma* 3.4 (ed. and trans. Bos, 14).

170. "Purple amaranth" (*yarbūz*): Note that Maimonides uses two different synonymous terms to indicate this plant, i.e., *baqla yamanīya* (cf. 20.47, 21.79) and *yarbūz*. See *Dioscurides triumphans* (ed. Dietrich, 2:100) and Maimonides, *Glossary of Drug Names*, no. 53 (ed. Rosner).

171. "craving for clay": On this phenomenon typical for pregnant women and called κίσσα (*pica*) in ancient sources, see Ibn al Jazzār, *On Sexual Diseases* 15 (pp. 180–89 [Arabic text], 285–88 [English translation]). Cf. also aphorism 16.23 above.

172. "turnips": The Arabic *saljam* is synonymous with *lift* and thus can mean both turnip and rape [*Brassica napus*]. Cf. Dioscurides, *Dioscurides Triumphans* 2.94 (ed. and trans. Dietrich, 2:257–59); and aphorisms 20.47, 72 above.

173. Īsā ibn Māssa was a medical author who was probably a contemporary of Ḥunayn ibn Isḥāq (ninth century). His otherwise unknown work, *Mirʾāt al-ṭibb*, is often quoted by al-Tamīmī (Ullmann, *Medizin im Islam*, 123).

174. "the smaller variety" (*khiyār*): Cf. Dioscurides, *Dioscurides triumphans* 4.173 (ed. and trans. Dietrich, 2:689–93, esp. 692 n. 14).

The Twenty-First Treatise

1. This text does not appear in the spurious edition edited by Kühn: Pseudo-Galen, *In Hippocratis De alimento commentarius* 4 (15:229–50). Cf. aphorism 16.32 above.

2. Cf. Galen, *De bonis malisque sucis* 2.5 (ed. Helmreich, 395, lines 10–11): καὶ διὰ τοῦτο τοῖς ἰατροῖς εὑρέθη τὰ κληθέντα πρὸς αὐτῶν ὑγιεινὰ φάρμακα (Therefore drugs have been invented by the physicians, which they called healthy).

3. Galen, *De bonis malisque sucis* 2.5 (ed. Helmreich, 395, lines 10–17).

4. "Astringent wine": I.e., sour, dry wine. Cf. Galen, *In Hippocratis De acutorum morborum victu commentarius* 3.8 (ed. Helmreich, 229, line 9): αὐστηρὸς.

5. "in that it": Lit. "and."

6. "suffering from a hot disease": I.e., having a fever. Cf. Galen, *In Hippocratis De acutorum morborum victu commentarius* 3.8 (ed. Helmreich, 229, line 13): τοῖς πυρέττουσιν.

7. Galen, *In Hippocratis De acutorum morborum victu commentarius* 3.8 (ed. Helmreich, 229, lines 8–9, 13–18).

8. Galen, *De sanitate tuenda* 4.4 (ed. Koch, 109, lines 4–6).

9. Galen, *De methodo medendi* 7.6 (ed. Kühn, 10:485; ed. and trans. Johnston and Horsley, 2:278–79).

10. "and expel them with the excrement": Lit. "and forward them to the excrement." Cf. Galen, *De methodo medendi* 7.6 (ed. Kühn, 10:486; ed. and trans. Johnston and Horsley, 2:280): καὶ τα περιττώματα πρὸς τὰς ἐκκρίσεις ποδηγοῦσι.

11. Galen, *In Hippocratis De acutorum morborum victu commentarius* 3.40 (ed. Helmreich, 253, lines 7–17; 254, lines 28–30).

12. Galen, *De victu attenuante* 6 (ed. Kalbfleisch, 439, lines 9–13).

13. "*sawīq*" (semolina): See Maimonides, *Glossary of Drug Names*, no. 284 (trans. Rosner): "It is wheat, barley and other similar roasted cereals, agitated with butter and then ground." See Galen, *De alimentorum facultatibus* 1.9.1 (ed. Helmreich, 228, line 24): ἄλφιτα (barley groats); see also Maimonides, *Medical Aphorisms* 5.16 (ed. and trans. Bos, 1:74).

14. "Even if its outer shell . . . suffer any harm from it": Galen, *De alimentorum facultatibus* 1.9.5 (ed. Helmreich, 230, lines 1–3).

15. "Because barley groats . . . mixed together": Galen, *De alimentorum facultatibus* 1.18.5 (ed. Helmreich, 244, lines 14–15).

16. Galen, *De alimentorum facultatibus* 3.14, 15; 3.15.1, 2 (ed. Helmreich, 349, lines 1–4, 10–14; 350, lines 4–8).

17. "solid, smooth stones": Cf. Galen, *De simplicium medicamentorum temperamentis ac facultatibus* 10.8 (ed. Kühn, 12:267): κάχληκας (pebbles).

18. "most of the moist, watery part" (i.e., the whey): Lit. "its watery part and most of its moisture." Cf. Galen, *De simplicium medicamentorum temperamentis ac facultatibus* 10.8 (ed. Kühn, 12:267): τὸ πλεῖστον ἐξ αὐτοῦ τῆς ὀρρώδους ὑγρότητος (most of the serum-like moisture).

19. "of oily things": Cf. Galen, *De simplicium medicamentorum temperamentis ac facultatibus* 10.8 (ed. Kühn, 12:267): δριμέων ῥευμάτων (of sharp liquids).

20. Galen, *De simplicium medicamentorum temperamentis ac facultatibus* 10.8 (ed. Kühn, 12:265, 267).

21. Galen, *De methodo medendi* 7.6 (ed. Kühn, 10:474–75; ed. and trans. Johnston and Horsley, 2:262–65).

22. "at certain intervals": Lit. "with long intervals." Cf. Galen, *De victu attenuante* 12 (ed. Kalbfleisch, 450, lines 25–26): ἔκ τινων διαστημάτων.

23. Galen, *De victu attenuante* 12 (ed. Kalbfleisch, 450, lines 24–26).

24. Galen, *De alimentorum facultatibus* 3.14.8 (ed. Helmreich, 347, lines 5–10).

25. Galen, *In Hippocratis De acutorum morborum victu commentarius* 3.2 (ed. Helmreich, 223, lines 1–4).

26. "Hydromel boiled with absinthe wormwood": Cf. Galen, *De methodo medendi* 7.11 (ed. Kühn, 10:517); English translation by Johnston and Horsley in *Method of Medicine*, 2:326–27: "It is suitable to drink melikraton provided the absinth is boiled on its own."

27. Galen, *De methodo medendi* 7.11 (ed. Kühn, 10:517; ed. and trans. Johnston and Horsley, 2:326–27).

28. Galen, *De victu attenuante* 12 (ed. Kalbfleisch, p. 450, line 37–p. 451, line 2).

29. Galen, *De simplicium medicamentorum temperamentis ac facultatibus* 10.10 (ed. Kühn, 12:273).

30. "rose oil": Cf. Galen, *De methodo medendi* 11.18 (ed. Kühn, 10:799): ῥοδίνον, and the translation by Johnston and Horsley in *Method of Medicine*, 3:206–7: "rosaceum." For its composition, see Dioscurides, *Pedanii Dioscuridis Anazarbei* 1.43 (ed. Wellmann, 1:42–43).

31. "If several days of the illness had already passed": Cf. Galen, *De methodo medendi* 11.18 (ed. Kühn, 10:799): ἐπὶ προήκοντι δὲ τῷ χρόνῳ, and the translation by Johnston and Horsley in *Method of Medicine*, 3:206–7: "at the appropriate time."

32. "thyme [*Thymus serpyllum* and var.]": Cf. Galen, *De methodo medendi* 11.18 (ed. Kühn, 10:799): σπονδυλίον και ἔρπυλλος, and the translation by Johnston and Horsley in *Method of Medicine*, 3:206–7: "spondylium and tufted thyme."

33. "because this drug weakens . . . hinder it": Cf. Galen, *De methodo medendi* 11.18 (ed. Kühn, 10:799): ὡς ἂν ἐκλυομένης αὐτῶν τῆς δυνάμεως ἐν τῷ μεταξὺ τεταγμένων ὀστῶν, and the translation by Johnston and Horsley, 3:206–7: "so that their potency is released in the interval between the relevant bones."

34. "castoreum": A desiccated excretion of the glands of the *Castor fiber* L.

35. Galen, *De methodo medendi* 11.18 (ed. Kühn, 10:799; ed. and trans. Johnston and Horsley, 3:206–9).

36. Galen, *In Hippocratis De acutorum morborum victu commentarius* 3.39 (ed. Helmreich, 251, lines 17–25).

37. Galen, *In Hippocratis De acutorum morborum victu commentarius* 3.28 (ed. Helmreich, 245, lines 17–25).

38. Galen, *In Hippocratis De acutorum morborum victu commentarius* 3.30, 31, 32 (ed. Helmreich, 246, lines 18–20; 247, lines 13–15, 25–29).

39. "three": Cf. Galen, *Puero epileptico consilium* 6 (ed. Keil, 19, line 16): "four" (τέταρτον).

40. "seven": Cf. Galen, *Puero epileptico consilium* 6 (ed. Keil, 19, line 18): "eight" (ὄγδοον).

41. Galen, *Puero epileptico consilium* 6 (ed. Keil, p. 19, line 16–p. 20, line 1).

42. This text has not been preserved in Kühn's fragmentary edition: Galen, *De victus ratione in morbis acutis secundum Hippocratem* (ed. Kühn, 19:182–221), but in the Arabic translation; see Galen, *On Regimen and Acute Diseases*, ed. and trans. Lyons, 80–81.

43. "[in the body]": Cf. Galen, *De victu attenuante* 12 (ed. Kalbfleisch, 450, line 15): ἐν τῷ σώματι.

44. Galen, *De victu attenuante* 12 (ed. Kalbfleisch, 450, lines 11–16).

45. "the different kinds of sandalwood": I.e., white, red, and yellow.

46. Galen, *De methodo medendi* 11.11 (ed. Kühn, 10:766; ed. and trans. Johnston and Horsley, 3:160–61).

47. *Galen, De methodo medendi* 10.9 (ed. Kühn, 10:701; ed. and trans. Johnston and Horsley, 3:60–63).

48. Galen, *De theriaca ad Pisonem* 4 (ed. Kühn, 14:225–26; ed. and trans. Richter-Bernburg, 109a [Arabic]; 64–65 [German]). Cf. aphorism 17.41 above.

49. Galen, *De theriaca ad Pisonem* 4 (ed. Kühn, 14:228; ed. and trans. Richter-Bernburg, 109b–110a [Arabic]; 66 [German]); cf. Anastassiou and Irmer, eds., *Testimonien zum Corpus Hippocraticum*, pt. 2, 2:165 (Hippocrates, *Deuxième Livre des Épidémies* 3.2 [ed. and trans. Littré 5:104, lines 6–12 (Greek), 105 (French)]).

50. Galen, *De victu attenuante* 4 (ed. Kalbfleisch, 436, lines 35–36; 437, lines 4–5, 7–8).

51. "medicine": In this context, "herb."

52. "neither thin [lit. "shriveled"] nor meager [lit. "emaciated"]": Cf. Galen, *De antidotis* 1.12 (ed. Kühn, 14:60): μὴ ῥυσὰ μηδὲ ἄτροφα (neither thin nor undernourished).

53. Galen, *De antidotis* 1.12 (ed. Kühn, 14:60).

54. Galen, *De antidotis* 1.5 (ed. Kühn, 14:31).

55. See the introduction to this volume.

56. Galen, *De bonis malisque sucis* 8.4 (ed. Helmreich, 415, lines 19–22).

57. "in the body": Galen, *In Hippocratis Epidemiarum librum 6 commentaria* 6 (ed. Wenkebach and trans. Pfaff, 344, lines 3–4) adds: as a result from a bad diet or pestilential air.

58. Galen, *In Hippocratis Epidemiarum librum 6 commentaria* 6 (ed. Wenkebach and trans. Pfaff, 344, lines 2–6; Latin in Deller, trans., "Exzerpta aus Epidemienkommentaren," 539 no. 91).

59. "that which": Cf. Galen, *De alimentorum facultatibus* 2.34.2 (ed. Helmreich, 302, line 11): φλέγμα (phlegm).

60. Galen, *De alimentorum facultatibus* 2.34.2 (ed. Helmreich, 302, lines 10–13).

61. "coagulated": Cf. Galen, *De sanitate tuenda* 4.5 (ed. Koch, 117, line 1): ἀργῶς συνεστῶτα.

62. Galen, *De sanitate tuenda* 4.5 (ed. Koch, p. 116, line 32–p. 17, line 2).

63. Galen, *De methodo medendi* 12.8 (ed. Kühn, 10:866; ed. and trans. Johnston and Horsley, 3:306–7).

64. "hard tumors": Cf. Galen, *De methodo medendi* 13.17 (ed. Kühn, 10:920): φλεγμονὴ; translation by Johnston and Horsley, 3:386–87: "inflammation."

65. "rustyback fern [or hart's tongue fern]": *Asplenium ceterach* or *Asplenium scolopendrium*. Cf. Maimonides, *Glossary of Drug Names*, no. 275 (trans. Rosner); and Dioscurides, *Dioscurides triumphans* 3.126 (ed. and trans. Dietrich, 2:488–89).

66. Galen, *De methodo medendi* 13.17 (ed. Kühn, 10:920–21; ed. and trans. Johnston and Horsley, 3:386–89).

67. Galen, *De compositione medicamentorum secundum locos* 4.5 (ed. Kühn, 12:720).

68. "putrefactive serous discharges": Cf. Galen, *De compositione medicamentorum secundum locos* 8.7 (ed. Kühn, 13:199): ἰχῶρας μοχθηροὺς.

69. "the [whole] class": Cf. Galen, *De compositione medicamentorum secundum locos* 8.7 (ed. Kühn, 13:199): ἅπαν γένος.

70. Galen, *De compositione medicamentorum secundum locos* 8.7 (ed. Kühn, 13:199–200).

71. Galen, *De compositione medicamentorum secundum locos* 8.7 (ed. Kühn, 13:130).

72. Galen, *De compositione medicamentorum secundum locos* 8.3 (ed. Kühn, 13:150).

73. Galen, *De compositione medicamentorum secundum locos* 8.7 (ed. Kühn, 13:201).

74. Galen, *De compositione medicamentorum secundum locos* 9.4 (ed. Kühn, 13:274–75).

75. "drugs that free [the body from poisons]": Or "drugs that save, i.e., antidotes." Cf. Galen, *De simplicium medicamentorum temperamentis ac facultatibus* 5.18 (ed. Kühn, 11:761): τὰς ἀλεξητηρίους τε καὶ ἀλεξιφαρμάκους ὀνομαζομένας δυνάμεις.

76. Galen, *De simplicium medicamentorum temperamentis ac facultatibus* 5.18 (ed. Kühn, 11:761, 763).

77. Galen, *De simplicium medicamentorum temperamentis ac facultatibus* 5.18 (ed. Kühn, 11:762–63).

78. Galen, *De antidotis* 1.15 (ed. Kühn, 14:91).

79. Galen, *De antidotis* (ed. Kühn, 14:92).

80. Galen, *De theriaca ad Pisonem* 14 (ed. Kühn, 14:270; ed. and trans. Richter-Bernburg, 123a–b [Arabic], 98 [German]).

81. Galen, *De theriaca ad Pisonem* 15 (ed. Kühn, 14:276–77; ed. and trans. Richter-Bernburg, 125a [Arabic], 102 [German]).

82. Galen, *De theriaca ad Pisonem* 16 (ed. Kühn, 14:280; ed. and trans. Richter-Bernburg, 126a [Arabic], 104 [German]).

83. **G** adds: "I do not advise you to administer the theriac in the summer or in a hot land. It should not be administered to a young person or to those suffering from heat, or, if we give [it to] them, it should only be a small amount. It should not at all be administered to boys because the strength of this drug is greater than the strength of their bodies, and one cannot be sure that it does not rapidly dissolve their bodies. A man once forced his son, while still a boy, to take this drug. It dissolved his body, made him suffer from diarrhea, and the boy died the following night." Cf. Galen, *De theriaca ad Pisonem* 17 (ed. Kühn, 14:285–87; ed. and trans. Richter-Bernburg, 127b–128a [Arabic], 108–9 [German]).

84. **Z** reads: "be-ᶜir Antokhia" (in the city of Antioch) and **Bo**: "in terris antiochie" (in the land of Antioch).

85. Pseudo-Galen, *De theriaca ad Pamphilianum* (ed. Kühn, 14:299). The literary title of this Pseudo-Galenic work as quoted by Maimonides is "The Treatise on the Preparation of the Theriac" (*Maqāla fī ᶜamal al-tiryāq*). It is usually referred to as *Kitāb al-tiryāq ilā Bamfūliyānūs* (Ullmann, *Medizin im Islam*, 49, no. 52). Ḥunayn ibn Isḥāq considered this work to be authentic—a rare mistake by him—and so it continued to be included among the genuine material by Galen. The inauthenticity was first suspected in the late sixteenth century and has been confirmed by modern research; see Nutton, "Galen on Theriac"; see also the introduction to this volume. The story quoted by Maimonides also shows up in the anonymous treatise on the plague entitled *Ha-maʾamar be-qaddahat ha-dever* (see Bos, "Black Death in Hebrew Literature").

86. Galen, *De theriaca ad Pisonem* 9 (ed. Kühn, 14:238; ed. and trans. Richter-Bernburg, 112b [Arabic], 73–74 [German]).

87. "weasel": Galen, *De theriaca ad Pisonem* 10 (ed. Kühn, 14:246): μυγαλῆ (shrew, field mouse); also see Richter-Bernburg's translation in "De Theriaca ad Pisonem," 115b (Arabic), 80, esp. n. 82 (German).

88. Cf. Galen, *De theriaca ad Pisonem* 10 (ed. Kühn, 14:246; ed. and trans. Richter-Bernburg, 115b [Arabic], 80 [German]).

89. Cf. Galen, *De theriaca ad Pisonem* 13 (ed. Kühn, 14:266; ed. and trans. Richter-Bernburg, 122b [Arabic], 96 [German]).

90. "heat": I.e., the heating effect of a remedy.

91. Galen, *De simplicium medicamentorum temperamentis ac facultatibus* 4 (ed. Kühn, 11:619–703). Maimonides' quotation seems to be a summary of disparate elements appearing throughout this text; see pp. 638, 646, 656, 682, 685, 695.

92. "pushes inwards": Cf. Galen, *De simplicium medicamentorum temperamentis ac facultatibus* 5.26 (ed. Kühn, 11:785): ἀποκρούεσθαι (to repel).

93. Cf. Galen, *De simplicium medicamentorum temperamentis ac facultatibus* 5.26 (ed. Kühn, 11:785–86).

94. Galen, *De simplicium medicamentorum temperamentis ac facultatibus* 4.17 (ed. Kühn, 11:679).

95. Galen, *De simplicium medicamentorum temperamentis ac facultatibus* 4.7 (ed. Kühn, 11:640).

96. "Anything that has . . . the stools": Cf. Galen, *De victu attenuante* 3 (ed. Kalbfleisch, 436, lines 4–6), English translation by Singer in *Galen: Selected Works*, 307–8: "Plants with an alkaline or salty taste have a certain cutting potential too; and most of these also purge the stomach."

97. Galen, *De victu attenuante* 3 (ed. Kalbfleisch, p. 435, line 32–p. 436, line 7).

98. "heating [power], but also drying [power]": Cf. Galen, *De simplicium medicamentorum temperamentis ac facultatibus* 4.19 (ed. Kühn, 11:685): οὐ θερμοὺς μόνον, ἀλλὰ καὶ ξηροὺς τὴν δύναμιν.

99. Cf. Galen, *De simplicium medicamentorum temperamentis ac facultatibus* 4.19 (ed. Kühn, 11:685).

100. "and thickened juice prepared from dried figs": Not in Galen, *De compositione medicamentorum secundum locos* 7.2 (ed. Kühn, 13:8).

101. "lily": The Arabic *sawsan* designates several species of Liliaceae and Iridaceae; in this case it is the blue lily (*Iris florentina*). Cf. Galen, *De compositione medicamentorum secundum locos* 7.2 (ed. Kühn, 13:8): ἴρις.

102. Galen, *De compositione medicamentorum secundum locos* 7.2 (ed. Kühn, 13:8).

103. "fine": Cf. Galen, *De simplicium medicamentorum temperamentis ac facultatibus* 5.19 (ed. Kühn, 11:765): λεπτομερῆ. For the meaning of this term in Galen's pharmacological works, see Debru, "Philosophie et pharmacologie."

104. Galen, *De simplicium medicamentorum temperamentis ac facultatibus* 5.19 (ed. Kühn, 11:764–65).

105. Galen, *De simplicium medicamentorum temperamentis ac facultatibus* 5.9 (ed. Kühn, 11:732).

106. "These kinds of remedies": I.e., that do dissolve and disperse.

107. "solid storax [*Styrax officinalis*]": I.e., *mayʿa [jāmida]*. Just like *lubnā*, *mayʿa* on its own can refer to both the liquid and the solid storax.

108. Galen, *De simplicium medicamentorum temperamentis ac facultatibus* 5.5.8 (ed. Kühn, 11:719, 728).

109. "carrot, wild carrot [*Daucus carota*] seed": *Daucus carota* is used for both wild and cultivated varieties of carrot. Cf. Maimonides, *Drug Names* (ed. Rosner), no. 94.

110. "valerian [possibly *Valeriana officinalis* and var.]": See Dietrich, ed. and trans., in Dioscurides, *Dioscurides triumphans* 1.8 (pp. 92–94).

111. "Jew's stone [*Lapis judaicus*]": I.e., the spine of a fossil echinid [*Cidaris glandiferus*], which originated in Syria and Palestine. Galen, *De simplicium medicamentorum temperamentis ac facultatibus* 5.13 (ed. Kühn, 11:748), reads: ὤχρα (ochre).

112. Galen, *De simplicium medicamentorum temperamentis ac facultatibus* 5.13 (ed. Kühn, 11:748–49).

113. "[because the type of drugs . . . development of milk]": Added following Galen, *De simplicium medicamentorum temperamentis ac facultatibus* 5.22 (ed. Kühn, 11:775): ὅσα μὲν γὰρ οὔτε ξηραίνει καὶ θερμαίνει μετρίως, εἰς γάλακτος γένεσιν χρηστά.

114. "a stronger heating effect": Lit. "a moderate heating effect," corrected to follow Galen, *De simplicium medicamentorum temperamentis ac facultatibus* 5.22 (ed. Kühn, 11:775): τὰ δ' ἐπὶ πλέον θερμαίμοντα.

115. Galen, *De simplicium medicamentorum temperamentis ac facultatibus* 5.22 (ed. Kühn, 11:775).

116. "the book [on drugs composed] by Ibn Wāfid": The *Kitāb al-adwiya al-mufrada*. Ibn Wāfid (999–1067), who served as a vizier in Toledo, also composed a book on compound medicines, entitled *Kitāb al-wisād fī l-ṭibb*; see the introduction to this volume. Ibn Wāfid was also a major source consulted by Maimonides for the explanation of the names of drugs in his *Glossary of Drug Names*; see Bos, "Maimonides' Medical Works and their Contributions," 251.

117. Ibn Sīnā (980–1037), the famous physician and philosopher, principally known for his *Kitāb al-qānūn fī al-ṭibb*. Maimonides consulted this work extensively for the composition of his *On Hemorrhoids* and also refers to it in *On Poisons* and *On Coitus*; see Bos, "Maimonides' Medical Works and their Contributions," 251. The statements by Freudenthal and Zonta, "Avicenna among Medieval Jews," 228, 273, that the reason "why Maimonides did not read Avicenna himself, especially the *Shifāʾ* and the *Canon*, remains a mystery," and that Maimonides is "a single, baffling exception" to the rule that "Jewish physicians used Avicenna's *Canon* extensively," should be revised in the light of these data.

118. "mace": The false aril of the nut of the nutmeg tree (*Myristica fragrans* Houtt.).

119. "manna": The sugary concretions on certain desert plants, especially diverse species of *Astragalus*. See Maimonides, *Glossary of Drug Names*, no. 386 (trans. Rosner).

120. Cf. Ibn Wāfid, *Kitāb al-adwiya al-mufrada*, 19–20.

121. "ivy [*Hedera helix*]": *Lablāb*. This term is originally a general term for all kinds of twining, climbing plants and then especially for ivy but also for bindweed [*Convolvulus arvensis*] and other species. Cf. *Wörterbuch der klassischen arabischen Sprache*, p. 2:93b, line 42–p. 94a, line 27.

122. "senna": For the numerous species of the senna (or cassia) legume, see Maimonides, *Glossary of Drug Names*, no. 267 (trans. Rosner).

123. "cardamom": I.e., a larger male variety [*Elettaria maior*], and a smaller female one, also called *ḥāl* [*Elettaria cardamomum*]; cf. Ibn Wāfid, *Kitāb al-adwiya al-mufrada*, 127–28.

124. "corundum" (*yāḳūt*): Cf. *Encyclopaedia of Islam*, new ed., s.v. "*yāḳūt*": "In medieval Arabic literary and scientific textual sources, *yāḳūt* is equivalent to all varieties of the mineral corundum that we know today. Corundum is a crystallised form of alumina ($A_{12}O_3$) that occurs in many colours, among which *yāḳūt aḥmar* ('red corundum' or 'ruby') is the finest."

125. "nard" (*sunbul*): The Arabic term is synonymous with *nārdīn*. For the main species see aphorism 17.39 above.

126. "labdanum": The resinous juice that exudes from *Cistus ladanifer, Cistus creticus, Cistus villosus,* and other species.

127. "mahaleb cherry [*Prunus mahaleb*]": Also called St. Lucie cherry.

128. "manna" (*mann*): The Arabic term is synonymous with *taranjubīn,* mentioned in aphorism 21.68 above. Cf. Maimonides, *Glossary of Drug Names,* no. 386 (trans. Rosner).

129. Cf. Ibn Wāfid, *Kitāb al-adwiya al-mufrada,* 20.

130. "*ṣeqāqul*": For its different species, all of which have an edible bulb, see Maimonides, *Glossary of Drug Names,* no. 361 (trans. Rosner).

131. Cf. Ibn Wāfid, *Kitāb al-adwiya al-mufrada,* 20.

132. "Indian and Chebulic [*Terminalia chebula* Retz] myrobalan": Indian or black myrobalan is the unripe fruit, while Chebulic myrobalan is the ripe fruit of *Terminalia chebula* Retz (Schmucker, *Pflanzliche und mineralische Materia medica,* no. 787).

133. "coral" (*bussad*): Originally, this term designated the root of the coral but was then used as a synonym of *marjān,* for coral itself. The Arabs took it for a plant that petrifies when one extracts it from the sea. Cf. *Encyclopaedia of Islam,* new ed., s.v. "*mardjān.*"

134. "sorrel, which is the same as wild beet": Cf. Maimonides, *Glossary of Drug Names,* no. 150 (trans. Rosner).

135. "mung bean": Cf. Ibn Janāḥ, *Kitāb al-Talkhīṣ* (forthcoming), no. 545:

الماش هو حبّ صغير، أصغر من اللوبياء وله عين كعين اللوبياء، وقد رأيتُه بقرطبة عند الوزير ابن شهيد، وكان يزرع في بعض (٥٠٥ آ) بساتينه وليس كان عند غيره بقرطبة، فأخبرني أنَّ ابن حسداي اليهودي كان جلبه إليه من المشرق.

(*Al-māṣ*) [mung bean] is a small seed, smaller than a black-eyed pea [*lūbiyā*]; it has an eye like that of the black-eyed pea. I have seen it in Córdoba at the abode of the vizier Ibn Ṣahīd. It was planted in one of his gardens; but it was not to be found at the abode of anyone else in Córdoba. He told me that Ibn Ḥasdāy, the Jew, had brought it to him from the East.)

136. "thistle" (*shukāʿā*): A general term for the different species of thistles. See Dioscurides, *Dioscurides triumphans* 3.13 (ed. and trans. Dietrich, 2:357–59); and Schmucker, *Pflanzliche und mineralische Materia medica,* no. 434.

137. "willow [*khilāf, Salix aegyptiaca*], which is identical with *al-ṣafṣāf*": Cf. Maimonides, *Glossary of Drug Names,* no. 393 (trans. Rosner). **ELO** add "emerald, pearl, haematite." Ibn Wāfid, *Kitāb al-adwiya al-mufrada,* 20, adds "glue."

138. Cf. Ibn Wāfid, *Kitāb al-adwiya al-mufrada,* 20.

139. Cf. Ibn Wāfid, *Kitāb al-adwiya al-mufrada,* 21.

140. "basil (which is the same as . . .)" (*faranjamushk*): The identity of the plant is uncertain; it is possibly *Ocimum basilicum* or *Ocimum minimum* or *Ocimum pilosum.* For other identifications see Maimonides, *Glossary of Drug Names,* no. 47 (trans. Rosner); Dioscurides, *Dioscurides triumphans* 3.43 (ed. and trans. Dietrich, 2:392–93); Schmucker, *Pflanzliche und mineralische Materia medica,* no. 529; and Ibn Wāfid, *Kitāb al-adwiya al-mufrada,* 58 (Spanish).

141. Cf. Ibn Janāḥ, *Kitāb al-Talkhīṣ* (forthcoming), no. 154: بَرَنْجَمُشْك هو الحبق

فوّاح ويتخذ منه دهن القرنفلي عن ابن جلجل وعن ابن الجزّار، وأخبرني أبو الفتوح أنّه ليس به بل هو من بقول المائدة، وهو بأن يغلّ في الشيرج، وقد ذكرنا قبل هذا قولَ أبي حنيفة فيه (*Baranjamushk* is the clove-like basil [*ḥabaq qaranfulī*], according to Ibn Juljul and Ibn al-Jazzār. Abū al-Futūḥ told me that this is not correct. It is rather a sort of vegetable served at the table. It is fragrant and a sort of aromatic oil can be made from it, if it is boiled in sesame oil [*shīraj*]. We have already quoted Abū Ḥanīfa's statement about this plant earlier.)

142. "bitumen of Judea [*kufr al-yahūd*], which is the same as *al-ḥumar*": Cf. Maimonides, *Glossary of Drug Names*, no. 168 (trans. Rosner); Schmucker, *Pflanzliche und mineralische Materia medica*, no. 586.

143. Cf. Ibn Janāḥ, *Kitāb al-Talkhīṣ* (forthcoming), no. 380: والحُمَر أيضًا هو قفر اليهود من كتاب العلل والأعراض (the term *ḥumar* stands also for Judean asphalt [*qufr al-Yahūd*], according to [Galen's] *Book on Causes and Symptoms* [*Kitāb al-ʿilal wa-l-aʿrāḍ*]).

144. "turnip": The Arabic term *lift* can also designate rape [*Brassica napus*]. See also aphorisms 20.47, 72, and 85 above.

145. "*falanja*": Cf. Maimonides, *Glossary of Drug Names*, no. 137 (trans. Rosner): "It is *al-falanja* and 'crow's foot' (*rijl al-ghurāb*) and 'grasshopper foot' (*rijl al-jirād*)." The identification of this plant is uncertain. For different suggestions, cf. Maimonides, *Glossary of Drug Names*, no. 137 (trans. Rosner) and Ibn Wāfid, *Kitāb al-adwiya al-mufrada*, 398 (Spanish translation). See as well Ibn Janāḥ, *Kitāb al-Talkhīṣ* (forthcoming), no. 317: زرنب هو فلنجة من الحاوي، وفي اللغة: زرنب هو فلنجة ضرب من الطيب (*Zarnab* is *falanja*, according to the *Ḥāwī*. From the lexicographical literature: *Zarnab* is *falanja*; it ranks among aromatic substances).

146. "narcissus": For the relevant different varieties, cf. Schmucker, *Pflanzliche und mineralische Materia medica*, no. 766; and Dioscurides, *Dioscurides triumphans* 4.147 (ed. and trans. Dietrich, 2:663).

147. "edible nut [i.e., walnut]" (*jawz al-maʾkūl*): Cf. Maimonides, *Glossary of Drug Names*, no. 82 (trans. Rosner); and Schmucker, *Pflanzliche und mineralische Materia medica*, no. 208.

148. "fenugreek [*Trigonella foenum graecum*]": **BG** read "flower of the wild pomegranate."

149. Cf. Ibn Wāfid, *Kitāb al-adwiya al-mufrada*, 21.

150. "behen (*bahman*)": The identification of this plant is uncertain. It may refer to *Centaurea behen* (a knapweed) or to a plant of the *Limonium* genus (statices or sea lavenders).

151. "wild senna [*Senna tora*] seed": For the doubtful identity of this plant, see Dioscurides, *Dioscurides triumphans* 3:121 (ed. and trans. Dietrich, 2:482–83).

152. "moghat [root of *Glossostemon Bruguieri* D.C., *mughādh*], which is the same as *mughāth*": This identification is the result of modern research undertaken by Schweinfurth. In medieval Arabic medical literature, the term is erroneously used for the rind of the root of the wild pomegranate tree; cf. Dioscurides, *Dioscurides triumphans* 1.82 (ed. and trans. Dietrich, 2:172n2); and Maimonides, *Glossary of Drug Names*, no. 219 (trans. Rosner). Ibn Wāfid, *Kitāb al-adwiya al-mufrada*, 412 (Spanish translation), has only the traditional medieval interpretation. For the term *moghat*, cf. Amin, Awad, Samad, and Iskander, "Isolation of Estrone." See also Ibn Janāḥ, *Kitāb al-Talkhīṣ* (forthcoming), no. 546: المغاذ هو عروق شجر الرمّان البرّي عن ابن الجزّار، وقال أبو حنيفة: أصل القلقل هو الذي يسمّيه الأطبّاء المغاذ، وإذا جُفّ ورقه وديف بالماء كان كالغِراء فيضمد به الخلع، وقال في القلقل شجيرة خضراء تنهض على ساق، ومنابتها الآكام دون الروض، ولها حبّ كحبّ اللوبياء حلو طيّب يؤكل، وقال أبو عمرو: القلقل من النبات الذي إذا جفّ ثمّ هبّ عليه الريح كان له جرس وزجل. (*Al-mughād* [gloss-ostemon] is the root of the wild pomegranate tree [*ʿurūq ajar al-rummān al-barrī*], according to Ibn al-Jazzār. Abū Ḥanīfa: *Ḥabb al-qilqil* is what the physicians call

al-muġāḏ. If its leaves are dried and mixed with water, a glue-like substance emerges, which can be applied to dislocations [*khalʿ*]. He said about *qilqil* [*Senna tora*]: It is a green shrub with an elevated stem; it grows on hills and not in gardens. It has a seed resembling that of the black-eyed pea [*lūbiyāʾ*], which is sweet, fragrant, and edible. Abū ʿAmr said: It is one of those plants that bring forth sounds and rattling noises when they have become dry and the wind touches them).

153. Cf. Ibn Wāfid, *Kitāb al-adwiya al-mufrada*, 21.

154. "gum tragacanth": From different *Astragalus* species. Cf. Maimonides, *Glossary of Drug Names*, no. 191 (trans. Rosner).

155. "waybread": Different *Plantago* species. Cf. Dioscurides, *Dioscurides triumphans* 2.108 (ed. and trans. Dietrich, 2:272–73).

156. "boxthorn" (*ʿawsaj*): The Arabic term is used for different species of *Lycium* but also of *Rhamnus* (buckthorns). Cf. Dioscurides, *Dioscurides triumphans* 1.59 (ed. and trans. Dietrich, 2:141–43); and Maimonides, *Glossary of Drug Names*, no. 294 (trans. Rosner).

157. Cf. Ibn Wāfid, *Kitāb al-adwiya al-mufrada*, 21.

158. "melon [*Cucumis melo*]": The Arabic term *bittīkh* also designates the watermelon [*Citrullus lanatus* var. *lanatus*], which is mentioned in this list under the name *dullāʿ*.

159. "[the smaller variety of] cucumber": See aphorism 20.87 above.

160. "gourd [pumpkin]": For different species, see Dioscurides, *Dioscurides triumphans* 2.116 (ed. and trans. Dietrich, 2:282); and Maimonides, *Glossary of Drug Names*, no. 332 (trans. Rosner).

161. Cf. Ibn Wāfid, *Kitāb al-adwiya al-mufrada*, 22.

162. **EGLO** add "pine resin" (of *Pinus sp.* and var.).

163. "wormwood [*Artemisia* spp.]" (*shīḥ*): The Arabic *shīḥ* is a general name for all *Artemisia* species and then perhaps especially for *Artemisia maritima*. See Dioscurides, *Dioscurides triumphans* 3.26 (ed. and trans. Dietrich, 2:371–72).

164. "oregano" (*ṣaʿtar*): Cf. aphorism 20.49 above.

165. "mint [*Mentha*]": For the different species, cf. *Encyclopaedia of Islam*, new ed., s.v. "*fūdhanj*."

166. "Ibn Sīnā says that it is [also] hot in the first degree": In the *Kitāb al-qānūn* 1.338, Ibn Sīnā remarks that it is *ḥār qalīl* (slightly hot) and dry in the second degree.

167. "*mūmiyā*": There are two kinds of '*mūmiyā*': the natural one, bitumen; and the human one, the bituminous mass of the Egyptian mummies. See Dioscurides, *Dioscurides triumphans* 1.39 (ed. and trans. Dietrich, 2:120–21); and also Maimonides, *Glossary of Drug Names*, no. 234 (trans. Rosner).

168. "*zarnab*": Its identity is uncertain; it has been identified with *Taxus baccata*, *Salix aegyptiaca*, and *Atriplex odorata*. Cf. Maimonides, *Glossary of Drug Names*, no. 137 (trans. Rosner); and Aguirre de Cárcer in Ibn Wāfid, *Kitāb al-adwiya al-mufrada*, 62n90 (Spanish translation).

169. "and some say that this is the same as *al-falanja*": See aphorism 21.75 above.

170. "grape ivy [*Rhoicissus rhomboidea*]": The identification of the Arabic term *ḥamāmā* with grape ivy is based on Ibn Sahl, *Dispensatorium parvum*, 241, 258; and Schmucker, *Pflanzlicher und mineralische Materia medica*, 258: "Weinartige

Klimmen." According to Dietrich in Dioscurides, *Dioscurides triumphans* 1.12 (ed. and trans. Dietrich, 2:98–99), an identification is impossible.

171. See treatise 20, n. 90.

172. Cf. Ibn Wāfid, *Kitāb al-adwiya al-mufrada*, 22.

173. "earth almonds [*ḥabb al-zalam, Cyperus esculentus*] (which are also called *ful-ful al-sudān*)": Cf. Dioscurides, *Dioscurides triumphans* 3.121 (ed. and trans. Dietrich, 2:482–83); and Maimonides, *Glossary of Drug Names*, no. 161 (trans. Rosner).

174. "thapsia [*Thapsia garganica, tāfsiyā*] (which is the same as *al-yantūn*)": Cf. Maimonides, *Glossary of Drug Names*, no. 380 (trans. Rosner); and Dioscurides, *Dioscurides triumphans* 4.142 (ed. and trans. Dietrich, 2:657–59).

175. Cf. Ibn Janāḥ, *Kitāb al-Talkhīṣ* (forthcoming), no. 433: البنتون هي التافسيا من الأدوية المفردة لجالينوس (*Yantūn* is *tāfsiyā*; from Galen's *Simple Drugs* [*Al-adwiyah al-mufradah*]).

176. Cf. Ibn Wāfid, *Kitāb al-adwiya al-mufrada*, 22.

177. "tabasheer": A white concretion obtained from the nodal joints of bamboo (*Bambusa bambos*).

178. "sandalwood": I.e., red [*Pterocarpus santalinus*] or white [*Santalum album*].

179. "dragon's blood [*dam al-akhawayn*, red resin of *Dracaena draco*], which is called *al-qāṭir* and also *al-shayyān*": Cf. Maimonides, *Glossary of Drug Names*, no. 96 (trans. Rosner).

180. Cf. Ibn Janāḥ, *Kitāb al-Talkhīṣ* (forthcoming), no. 73: الأيْدَع الشَيّان، وقال أبو حنيفة: أخبرني أعرابي أنّه صمغ أحمر يؤتى به من سقطرى جزيرة الصَّبِر، تداوى به الجراحات، وقال آخر: بل هو شجر أحمر يُصبَغ به، وهو عند الرواة دم الأخوَين (*Al-aydaʿ* is the houseleek [*shayyān*]. Abū Ḥanīfa: A Bedouin told me that it is a red resin imported from Socotra, the island of aloe. It is used for the treatment of injuries. Someone else told me that it is a red tree that is used for dyeing. According to the narrators [of ancient poetry], it is dragon's blood [*dam al-akhawayn*]).

181. Cf. Ibn Wāfid, *Kitāb al-adwiya al-mufrada*, 22.

182. "knotgrass [*ʿaṣā al-rāʿī, Polygonum aviculare*], which is called *al-qaḍāb* in Egypt": Cf. Schmucker, *Pflanzliche und mineralische Materia medica*, no. 430.

183. Cf. Ibn Wāfid, *Kitāb al-adwiya al-mufrada*, 22–23.

184. "*kundus*": Cf. *Wörterbuch der klassischen arabischen Sprache*, 1:379a lines 29–36: "sneezewort (*Achillea Ptarmica* L.), [. . .] also soap-wort, fuller's herb (*Saponaria officinalis* L.) [. . .] and gypsophila (species of *Gypsophila*), the various roots of which contain saponin."

185. "mezereon [*Daphne mesereum*]": Or perhaps *Daphne oleoides*.

186. "pepperweed [*Lepidium latifolium*]": The term *ṣīṭaraj* normally refers to the garden cress [*Lepidium sativum L.*]. It was, notwithstanding, also applied to other plants, especially the common leadwort [*Plumbago europaea*] or the pepperweed. See Maimonides, *Glossary of Drug Names*, no. 367 (ed. Rosner).

187. "spurge [*farbiyūn, Euphorbia resinifera* and var.] (which is the same as *al-tākūt*)": Cf. Maimonides, *Glossary of Drug Names*, no. 25 (trans. Rosner).

188. "leek (which has varieties)": Cf. Maimonides, *Glossary of Drug Names*, no. 198 (trans. Rosner).

189. "Poppy": Cf. Ibn Wāfid, *Kitāb al-adwiya al-mufrada*, 23.

190. "the different kinds of earth": E.g., sigillate earth, Armenian earth, Samian earth. Cf. Maimonides, *Glossary of Drug Names*, no. 172 (trans. Rosner).

191. "vitriol in its different types": Cf. Maimonides, *Glossary of Drug Names*, no. 140 (trans. Rosner).

192. "The color of natural bile": Lit. "the natural color of bile."

193. Galen, *De simplicium medicamentorum temperamentis ac facultatibus* 10.2 (ed. Kühn, 12:275–76).

194. Galen, *De simplicium medicamentorum temperamentis ac facultatibus* 10.2 (ed. Kühn, 12:280).

195. "of chickens": Cf. Galen, *De simplicium medicamentorum temperamentis ac facultatibus* 10.2 (ed. Kühn, 12:280): περδίκων (of partridges).

196. "more proper": Cf. Galen, *De simplicium medicamentorum temperamentis ac facultatibus* 10.2 (ed. Kühn, 12:280): ἀρείνους.

197. Cf. Galen, *De simplicium medicamentorum temperamentis ac facultatibus* 10.2 (ed. Kühn, 12:280).

198. Galen, *De methodo medendi* 6.2 (ed. Kühn, 10:392; ed. and trans. Johnston and Horsley, 2:128–29).

199. "three parts": Cf. Galen, *De methodo medendi* 10.4 (ed. Kühn, 10:703): τριπλάσιον ἢ τετραπλάσιον; translation by Johnston and Horsley, *Method of Medicine*, 3:64–65: "three or four parts."

200. "[rose] oil": Cf. Galen, *De methodo medendi* 10.4 (ed. Kühn, 10:703; ed. and trans. Johnston and Horsley, 3:64): τὸ ῥόδινον.

201. "is softened": Galen, *De methodo medendi* 10.4 (ed. Kühn, 10:703) adds ἐν θυείᾳ; translation by Johnston and Horsley, *Method of Medicine*, 3:64–65: "in a mortar."

202. "a *dabīqī* cloth": Dabīq was a locality in the outer suburbs of Damietta, noted for the manufacture of high-quality woven material that was to become so well known that the word came to designate a type of material. Cf. *Encyclopaedia of Islam*, new ed., s.v. "*Dabīḳ*"; and also Galen, *De methodo medendi* 10.4 (ed. Kühn, 10:703): ὀθόνιον δίπτυχον; translation by Johnston and Horsley, *Method of Medicine*, 3:64–65: "double thickness linen."

203. "*sawīq*" (semolina): Cf. Maimonides, *Glossary of Drug Names*, no. 284 (trans. Rosner): "It is wheat, barley and other similar roasted cereals, agitated with butter and then ground"; and Galen, *In Hippocratis Epidemiarum librum 6 commentaria* 6 (CMG 5.10.2.2; ed. Wenkebach and trans. Pfaff, 342, line 12; 343, line 6): κυκεών; see also aphorism 21.9 above.

204. Galen, *De methodo medendi* 10.4 (ed. Kühn, 10:703; ed. and trans. Johnston and Horsley, 3:64–65).

205. "[Pains of the eyes . . . be soothed]": Cf. Galen, *De methodo medendi* 12.8 (ed. Kühn, 10:867): τὰ τῶν ὀφθαλμῶν καὶ τὰ τῶν ὤτων ἀλγήματα διὰ τοιοῦτον χυμὸν ἢ πνεῦμα φυσῶδες ἐν πυρτοῖς γινόμενα πραΰνειν προσήκει; translation by Johnston and Horsley, *Method of Medicine*, 3:309: "[. . .] it is appropriate to soothe the pains of the eyes and ears that occur due to such a humor or vaporous *pneuma* in fevers."

206. Galen, *De methodo medendi* 12.8 (ed. Kühn, 10:867; ed. and trans. Johnston and Horsley, 3:308–9).

207. Galen, *Ad Glauconem de methodo medendi* 2.9 (ed. Kühn, 11:118–19).

208. "Al-Tamīmī says in his [book entitled] *Al-murshid*": See aphorism 19.82 above.

209. "*mithqāl*": 4.46 grams.

210. "quince juice" (*maybih*): Cf. Dozy, *Supplément aux dictionnaires arabes*, 2:635a, s.v. مِيبة: "(pers. مي به, 'vin de coings'): eau de coings, faite de vin et de jus de coings avec du sucre."

Bibliographies

Translations and Editions of Works by or Attributed to Moses Maimonides

(arranged alphabetically by translator or editor)

Bar-Sela, Ariel, Hebbel E. Hoff, and Elias Faris, eds. and trans. *Moses Maimonides' Two Treatises on the Regimen of Health: "Fī tadbīr al-ṣiḥḥah" and "Maqālah fī bayān baʿḍ al-aʿraḍ wa-al-jawāb ʿanhā."* Philadelphia: American Philosophical Society, 1964.

Barzel, Uriel S., ed. and trans. *The Art of Cure: Extracts from Galen.* Foreword by Fred Rosner; bibliography by Jacob I. Dienstag. Haifa: Maimonides Research Institute, 1992.

Bos, Gerrit, ed. and trans. *Commentary on Hippocrates' Aphorisms.* Provo, UT: Brigham Young University Press, forthcoming.

———, ed. and trans. *Medical Aphorisms.* 7 vols. Provo, UT: Brigham Young University Press, 2004–.

———, ed. and trans. *On Asthma.* Provo, UT: Brigham Young University Press, 2002.

———, ed. and trans. *On the Elucidation of Some Symptoms and the Response to Them.* Provo, UT: Brigham Young University Press, forthcoming.

Bos, Gerrit, ed. and trans., and Charles Burnett, ed. *On Coitus.* Including an edition and translation of the medieval Slavonic text by Will Ryan and Moshe Taube. Provo, UT: Brigham Young University Press, forthcoming.

Bos, Gerrit, ed. and trans., and Michael R. McVaugh, ed. *On Asthma, Volume 2.* Provo, UT: Brigham Young University Press, 2008.

Bos, Gerrit, ed. and trans., and Michael R. McVaugh, ed. *On Hemorrhoids.* Provo, UT: Brigham Young University Press, 2012.

Bos, Gerrit, ed. and trans., and Michael R. McVaugh, ed. *On Poisons and the Protection against Lethal Drugs.* Provo, UT: Brigham Young University Press, 2009.

Bos, Gerrit, ed. and trans., and Michael R. McVaugh, ed. *The Regimen of Health.* Provo, UT: Brigham Young University Press, forthcoming.

Deller, K. H., ed. and trans., and K. Deichgräber, ed. "Die Exzerpte des Moses Maimonides aus den Epidemienkommentaren des Galen." Supplement to Galen, *In*

Hippocratis Epidemiarum librum VI commentaria I–VIII, edited by Ernst Wenkebach and Franz Pfaff. CMG 5.10.2.2. Berlin: Akademie Verlag, 1956.

Efros, Israel, ed. and trans. *Maimonides' Treatise on Logic (Maḳālah fi-ṣināʿat al-manṭiḳ): The Original Arabic and Three Hebrew Translations.* New York: American Academy for Jewish Research, 1938.

Kroner, Hermann, ed. "Der medizinische Schwanengesang des Maimonides: *Fī bajān al-aʿrāḍ (Über die Erklärung der Zufälle)." Janus* 32 (1928): 12–116.

Meyerhof, Max, ed. and trans. *Sharḥ asmāʾ al-ʿuqqār/L'explication des noms des drogues: Un glossaire de matière médicale composé par Maïmonide.* Cairo: Imprimerie de l'Institut français d'archéologie orientale, 1940. See also Rosner's translation below.

Muntner, Süssman, ed. *Pirḳe Mosheh bi-refuʾah.* Jerusalem: Mosad ha-Rav Ḳuḳ, 1959.

Rosner, Fred, trans. *The Medical Aphorisms of Moses Maimonides.* Haifa: Maimonides Research Institute, 1989.

———, trans. *Moses Maimonides' Glossary of Drug Names.* Haifa: Maimonides Research Institute, 1995. See also Meyerhof's edition and translation above.

Stern, Samuel Miklos, ed. and trans. "Maimonides' *Treatise to a Prince, Containing Advice on Sexual Matters.*" In *Maimonidis Commentarius in Mischnam e codibus Hunt, 117 et Pococke 295 in Bibliotheca Bodleiana Oxoniensi servatis et 72–73 Bibliothecae Sassooniensis Letchworth*, edited by Samuel Miklos Stern, 17–21. Copenhagen: Ejnar Munksgaard, 1956–66.

Editions of Galenic Works

(arranged alphabetically by translator or editor)

Boer, Wilko de, ed. *Galeni de propriorum animi cuiuslibet affectuum dignotione et curatione, de animi cuiuslibet peccatorum dignotione et curatione, de atra bile.* CMG 5.4.1.1. Leipzig: Teubner, 1937.

Boudon-Millot, Véronique, ed. and trans. *Exhortation à l'étude de la médecine: Art médical.* Vol. 2 of *Galien.* Paris: Belles Lettres, 2000.

Brock, Arthur John, trans. *On the Natural Faculties.* 1916. Reprint, Cambridge, MA: Harvard University Press, 1979.

De Lacy, Phillip, ed. and trans. *On Semen.* CMG 5.3.1. Berlin: Akademie Verlag, 1992.

Grant, Mark, trans. *Galen on Food and Diet.* London: Routledge, 2000. See also Helmreich's edition below.

Green, Robert Montraville, trans. *A Translation of Galen's "Hygiene" (De sanitate tuenda).* Introduction by Henry E. Sigerist. Springfield, IL: Thomas, 1951. See also Koch's edition below.

Helmreich, Georg, ed. *De alimentorum facultatibus.* CMG 5.4.2. Leipzig: Teubner, 1923. See also Grant's translation above.

———, ed. *De bonis malisque sucis.* CMG 5.4.2. Leipzig: Teubner, 1923.

———, ed. *De usu partium corporis humani.* 2 vols. Bibliotheca Scriptorum Graecorum et Romanorum Teubneriana. 1907–9. Reprint, Amsterdam: Adolf M. Hakkert, 1968. See also May's translation below.

————,ed. *In Hippocratis de victu acutorum commentaria*. CMG 5.9.1. Leipzig: Teubner, 1914.

Johnston, Ian, and G. H. R. Horsley, eds. and trans. *Method of Medicine*. 3 vols. Harvard: Loeb Classical Library, 2011.

Kalbfleisch, Karl, ed. *De victu attenuante*. CMG 5.4.2. Leipzig: Teubner, 1923.

Keil, Winfried, ed. and trans. "Galeni *Puero epileptico consilium*: Ausgabe und kommentar." PhD diss., University of Göttingen, 1959.

Klein-Franke, Felix, ed. and trans. "The Arabic Version of Galen's Περὶ ἐθῶν." *Jerusalem Studies in Arabic and Islam* 1 (1979): 125–50.

Koch, Konrad, ed. *De sanitate tuenda*. CMG 5.4.2. Leipzig: Teubner, 1923. See also Green's translation above.

Kühn, Karl Gottlob, ed. *Claudii Galeni opera omnia*. 20 vols. 1821–33. Reprint, Hildesheim, Germany: Georg Olms, 1964–65.

Lyons, Malcolm, ed. and trans. *On the Parts of Medicine. On Cohesive Causes. On Regimen in Acute Diseases in Accordance with the Theories of Hippocrates*. CMG Suppl. Orient. 2. Berlin: Akademie Verlag, 1969.

May, Margaret Tallmadge, trans. *Galen on the Usefulness of the Parts of the Body*. 2 vols. Ithaca, NY: Cornell University Press, 1968. See also Helmreich's edition above.

Mewaldt, Johannes, ed. *In Hippocratis De natura hominis commentaria tria*. CMG 5.9.1. Leipzig: Teubner, 1914.

Nabielek, R., ed. and trans. "Die ps.-galenische Schrift *Über Schlaf und Wachsein* zum ersten Male herausgegeben, übersetzt und erläutert." PhD diss., Humboldt-Universität zu Berlin, 1977.

Richter-Bernburg, Lutz, ed. and trans. "Eine arabische Version der pseudogalenischen Schrift *De Theriaca ad Pisonem*." PhD diss., University of Göttingen, 1969.

Savage-Smith, Emilie, ed. and trans. "Galen on Nerves, Veins and Arteries." PhD diss., University of Wisconson, 1969.

Schmutte, Joseph M., ed. *Galeni de consuetudinibus*. With a German translation of Hunayn's Arabic version by Franz Pfaff. CMG, Supplement 3. Leipzig: Teubner, 1941.

Siegel, Rudolph E., trans. *Galen on the Affected Parts: Translation from the Greek Text with Explanatory Notes*. New York: Karger, 1976.

Singer, Peter N., trans. *Galen: Selected Works*. New York: Oxford University Press, 1997.

Wasserstein, Abraham, ed. and trans. *Galen's Commentary on the Hippocratic Treatise "Airs, Waters, Places": In the Hebrew Translation of Solomon ha-Meʾati*. Jerusalem: Israel Academy of Sciences and Humanities, 1983.

Wenkebach, Ernst, ed., and Franz Pfaff, trans. *Galeni in Hippocratis Epidemiarum libros I et II (III, VI commentaria)*. CMG 5.10.1. Leipzig: Teubner, 1934.

Wenkebach, Ernst, ed., and Franz Pfaff, trans. *Galeni in Hippocratis Epidemiarum librum III* CMG 5.10.2.1. Leipzig and Berlin: Teubner-Akademie Verlag, 1936.

Wenkebach, Ernst, ed., and Franz Pfaff, trans. *Galeni in Hippocratis Epidemiarum librum VI commentaria I–VIII*. CMG 5.10.2.2. Berlin: Academiae Litterarum, 1956.

General Bibliography

Álvarez Millán, Cristina. "Actualización del corpus médico-literario de los Banū Zuhr: Nota bibliográfica." *Al-qanṭara: Revista de estudios árabes* 16, no.1 (1995): 173–80.

Amin, El S., Olfat Awad, M. Abd El Samad, and M. N. Iskander. "Isolation of Estrone from *Moghat* Roots and from Pollen Grains of Egyptian Date Palm." *Phytochemistry* 8, no. 1 (1969): 295–97.

Anastassiou, Anargyros, and Dieter Irmer, eds. *Testimonien zum Corpus Hippocraticum*. Part 2, Galen. 2 vols. Göttingen, Germany: Vandenhoeck and Ruprecht, 1997, 2001.

Aristotle. *Aristotle's "De anima" Translated into Hebrew by Zeraḥyah ben Isaac ben She'altiel Ḥen: A Critical Edition with an Introduction and Index*. Edited by Gerrit Bos. Leiden: Brill, 1994.

Baron, Salo Wittmayer. *A Social and Religious History of the Jews*. Vol. 8, *High Middle Ages, 500–1200: Philosophy and Science*. 2nd ed. New York: Columbia University Press, 1952–83.

Beit-Arié, Malachi, comp., and R. A. May, ed. *Catalogue of the Hebrew Manuscripts in the Bodleian Library: Supplement of Addenda and Corrigenda to Vol. 1 (A. Neubauer's Catalogue)*. Oxford: Clarendon, 1994. See also Neubauer's catalogue below.

Blau, Joshua. *The Emergence and Linguistic Background of Judaeo-Arabic: A Study of the Origins of Middle Arabic*. London: Oxford University Press, 1965. Reprint, Jerusalem: Ben Zvi Institute for the Study of Jewish Communities in the East, 1981.

Bos, Gerrit. "Maimonides' Medical Aphorisms: Towards a Critical Edition and Revised English Translation." *Ḳorot* 12 (1996–97): 35–79.

———. "Maimonides' Medical Works and Their Contributions to His Medical Biography." *Maimonidean Studies* 5 (2008): 243–66.

———. "Maimonides on the Preservation of Health." *Journal of the Royal Asiatic Society. Third Series* 4, no. 2 (1994): 213–35.

———. *Novel Medical and General Hebrew Terminology from the 13th Century*. 2 vols. Oxford: Oxford University Press, 2011, 2013.

———, ed. and trans. "The Black Death in Hebrew Literature: *Ha-Ma'amar be-qaddaḥat ha-dever* (*Treatise on Pestilential Fever*)." *European Journal of Jewish Studies* 5, no. 1 (2011): 1–52.

Bustānī, Buṭrus, al-. *Kitāb muḥīṭ al-muḥīṭ*. 2 vols. Beirut, 1867–69.

Cano Ledesma, Aurora. *Indización de los manuscritos árabes de El Escorial*. Madrid: Ediciones Escurialenses, Real Monasterio de El Escorial, 1996.

Colin, Gabriel. *Avenzoar: Sa vie et ses oeuvres*. Paris: Leroux, 1911.

Debru, Armelle. "Philosophie et pharmacologie: La dynamique des substances leptomères chez Galien." In *Galen on Pharmacology: Philosophy, History and Medicine*, edited by Armelle Debru, 85–102. Leiden: Brill, 1997.

Derenbourg, Hartwig, comp. *Médecine et histoire naturelle*. Vol. 2, fasc. 2 of *Les manuscrits arabes de l'Escorial*. Revised and completed by H. P. J. Renaud. Paris: Librairie Orientaliste Paul Geuthner, 1941.

Dioscurides. *Des Pedanios Dioskurides aus Anazarbos: Arzneimittellehre in fünf Büchern.* Edited and translated by Julius Berendes. 1902. Reprint, 1 vol., Wiesbaden: Dr. Martin Sändig, 1970.

———. *Dioscurides triumphans: Ein anonymer arabischer Kommentar (Ende 12. Jahrh. n. Chr.) zur Materia medica.* Edited and translated by Albert Dietrich. 2 vols. Göttingen: Vandenhoeck and Ruprecht, 1988.

———. *Pedanii Dioscuridis Anazarbei De materia medica, libri quinque.* Edited by Max Wellmann. 3 vols. 5 bks. 1906–14. Reprint, in 1 vol., Berlin: Weidmann, 1958.

Dozy, Reinhart Pieter Anne. *Supplément aux dictionnaires arabes.* 2 vols. 2nd ed. Leiden: Brill, 1927.

Encyclopaedia of Islam. New edition. 12 vols. Leiden: Brill, 1960–94.

Endress, Gerhard, and Dimitri Gutas, eds. *A Greek and Arabic Lexicon (GALex): Materials for a Dictionary of the Mediaeval Translations from Greek into Arabic.* Fasc. 1ff. Leiden: Brill, 1992–.

Freudenthal, Gad. "Les sciences dans les communautés juives médiévales de Provence: Leur appropriation, leur rôle." *Revue des études juives,* vol. 152, fasc. 1–2 (1993): 29–136.

Freudenthal, Gad, and Mauro Zonta. "Avicenna among Medieval Jews. The Reception of Avicenna's Philosophical, Scientific and Medical Writings in Jewish Cultures, East and West." *Arabic Sciences and Philosophy* 22 (2012): 217–87.

Friedenwald, Harry. *The Jews and Medicine: Essays.* 2 vols. 1944. Reprint, New York: Ktav, 1967.

Giunta, Tomaso, ed. *De balneis: Omnia quae extant apud Graecos, Latinos, et Arabas, tam medicos quam quoscunque caeterarum artium probatos scriptores . . .* Venice: Giunta, 1553.

Hippocrates. *Epidemics 1 and 3.* In *Hippocrates: Volume 1*, edited and translated by W. H. S. Jones, 139–288. Loeb Classical Library 147. Cambridge, MA: Harvard University Press, 1923.

———. *Epidemics 2, 4–7.* In *Hippocrates: Volume 7*, edited and translated by Wesley D. Smith. Loeb Classical Library 477. Cambridge, MA: Harvard University Press, 1994.

———. *Œuvres complètes d'Hippocrate.* Edited and translated by É. Littré. 10 vols. 1839–61. Reprint, Amsterdam: Hakkert, 1973–82.

Hopkins, Simon. "The Language of Maimonides." In *The Trias of Maimonides: Jewish, Arabic, and Ancient Culture of Knowledge/Die Trias des Maimonides: Jüdische, arabische und antike Wissenskultur.* Edited by Georges Tamer, 85–106. New York: de Gruyter, 2005.

Ibn Abī Uṣaybiʿah. *ʿUyūn al-anbāʾ fī ṭabaqāt al-aṭibbāʾ.* Edited by Nizār Riḍā. Beirut: Dār Maktabat al-Ḥayah, 1965.

Ibn al-Jazzār. *Ibn al-Jazzār on Sexual Diseases and Their Treatment: A Critical Edition, English Translation, and Introduction of Book 6 of "Zād al musāfir wa-qūt al-ḥāḍir."* Edited and translated by Gerrit Bos. New York: Kegan Paul International, 1997.

Ibn al-Nadīm. *Kitāb al-fihrist.* Cairo: Miṭbaʿa al-istiqāma, 1928.

Ign al-Tilmīd, Hibat Allāh ibn Ṣāʿid. *The Dispensatory of Ibn at-Tilmīd.* Edited and translated by Oliver Kahl. Leiden: Brill, 2007.

Ibn Ezra, Abraham. *Sefer Hanisyonot: The Book of Medical Experiences attributed to Abraham ibn Ezra.* Edited, translated, and commented on by Joshua O. Leibowitz and Shlomo Marcus. Jerusalem: Magnes Press, 1984.

Ibn Isḥāq, Ḥunayn. *Ḥunain ibn Isḥāq über die syrischen und arabischen Galen-Übersetzungen: Zum ersten Mal herausgegeben und übersetzt.* Edited by Gotthelf Bergsträsser. Leipzig: Brockhaus, 1925.

Ibn Janāḥ, Abū al-Walīd Marwān. *Kitāb al-Talkhīṣ.* Edited and translated by Gerrit Bos, Fabian Käs, Guido Mensching, and Mailyn Lübke, forthcoming.

Ibn Sahl. *Dispensatorium parvum (al-Aqrābādhīn al-ṣaghīr).* Edited by Oliver Kahl. Leiden: Brill, 1994.

Ibn Sīnā. *Kitāb al-qānūn fī al-ṭibb.* 5 bks. in 3 vols. 1877. Reprint, Beirut: Dār Ṣādir, n.d.

Ibn Wāfid. *Kitāb al-adwiya al-mufrada (Libro de los Medicamentos Simples).* Edited and translated by Luisa Fernanda Aguirre de Cárcer. 2 vols. (vol.1: Spanish translation; vol. 2: Arabic text). Madrid: Consejo Superior de Investigaciones Científicas, Agencia Española de Cooperación Internacional, 1995.

———. *Kitāb al-wisād fī l-ṭibb (Libro de la Almohada, Sobre Medicina).* Edited and translated by Camilo Álvarez de Morales y Ruiz-Matas. Toledo: Diputación de Toledo, 2006.

Ibn Zuhr, Abū al-ꜥAlāʾ. *La Teḍkira d'Abū ʾl-ꜥAlāʾ.* Edited and translated by Gabriel Colin. Paris: Ernest Leroux, 1911.

Ibn Zuhr, Abū Marwān. *Kitāb al-agḍhiya (Tratado de los Alimentos).* Edited and translated by Expiración García Sánchez. Madrid: Consejo Superior de Investigaciones Científicas, Instituto de Cooperación con el Mundo Árabe, 1992.

Issa, Ahmed. *Dictionaire des Noms des Plantes en Latin, Français, Anglais et Arabe.* Cairo: Imprimerie Nationale, 1930.

Kahle, Paul. "Mosis Maimonidis Aphorismorum praefatio et excerpta." Appendix 2 of *Galeni in Platonis Timaeum commentarii fragmenta*, edited by Heinrich Otto Schröder, 89–99. CMG, Supplement 1. Leipzig: Teubner, 1934.

Kaufmann, David. "Le neveu de Maïmonide." *Revue des études juives* 7 (1883): 152–53.

Kohen, Solomon ben Abraham ha-. *Sheʾelot u-Teshuvot.* Vol. 2. Venice: 1592.

Kraemer, Joel L. "Six Unpublished Maimonides Letters from the Cairo Genizah." *Maimonidean Studies* 2, no. 1 (1991): 61–94.

Kuhne Brabant, Rosa. "Abū Marwān b. Zuhr: Un professionel de la médecine en plein XIIème siècle." In *Actes du VII Colloque universitaire tuniso-espagnol sur le patrimoine andalous dans la culture arabe et espagnole, Tunis, 3–10 février 1989,* 129–41. Tunis: Université de Tunis, Centre d'études et de recherches économiques et sociales, 1991.

Lane, Edward William. *Arabic-English Lexicon.* 8 vols. London: Williams and Norgate, 1863–93.

Langermann, Y. Tzvi. "Arabic Writings in Hebrew Manuscripts: A Preliminary Listing." *Arabic Sciences and Philosophy* 6, no. 1 (1996): 137–60.

———. "Gersonides on the Magnet and the Heat of the Sun." In *Studies on Gersonides: A Fourteenth-Century Jewish Philosopher-Scientist,* edited by Gad Freudenthal, 267–84. Leiden: Brill, 1992.

Leclerc, Lucien. *Histoire de la médecine arabe.* 2 vols. Paris: Ernest Leroux, 1876.

Levinger, Jacob. "Maimonides' *Guide of the Perplexed* on Forbidden Food in the Light of His Own Medical Opinion." In *Perspectives on Maimonides: Philosophical and Historical Studies*, edited by Joel L. Kraemer, 195–208. Littman Library. Oxford: Oxford University Press, 1991.

Liddell, H. G., and R. Scott. *A Greek-English Lexicon*. Revised and augmented throughout by H. S. Jones et al. 9th ed. With a supplement, 1968. Reprint, Oxford: Clarendon Press, 1989.

Lieber, Elinor. "Maimonides, the Medical Humanist." *Maimonidean Studies* 4 (2000): 39–60.

Meyerhof, Max. "The Medical Work of Maimonides." In *Essays on Maimonides: An Octocentennial Volume*, edited by Salo Wittmayer Baron, 265–99. New York: Columbia University Press, 1941.

———. "Über echte und unechte Schriften Galens, nach arabischen Quellen." *Sitzungsberichte der Preußischen Akademie der Wissenschaften zu Berlin: Philosophisch-historischen Klasse* 28 (1928): 533–48.

Neubauer, Adolf. *Catalogue of the Hebrew Manuscripts in the Bodleian Library and in the College Libraries of Oxford*. 2 vols. 1886–1906. Reprint, Oxford: Clarendon, 1994. See also Beit-Arié's supplement above.

Nutton, Vivian. "Galen on Theriac: Problems of Authenticity." In *Galen on Pharmacology: Philosophy, History and Medicine*, edited by Armelle Debru, 133–51. Leiden: Brill, 1997.

Oribasius. *Collectiones medicae*. Edited by Johann Raeder. CMG 6.1–2. 4 vols. Leipzig: Teubner, 1928–33.

Pertsch, Wilhelm. *Die arabischen Handschriften der herzoglichen Bibliothek zu Gotha*. Vol. 4, pt. 3, *Die Orientalischen Handschriften der herzoglichen Bibliothek zu Gotha*. Gotha, Germany: Perthes, 1877–92.

Ravitzky, Aviezer. "Mishnato shel Rabi Zeraḥyah ben Yitshak ben Sheᶜaltiʾel Ḥen wehe-hagut ha-maimonit-tibonit ba-meʾah ha-13." PhD diss., Hebrew University, 1977.

Rāzī, Abū Bakr Muḥammad ibn Zakariyā al-. *Kitāb al-ḥāwī fī al-ṭibb*. Vols. 1–23. Hyderabad, India: Daʾiratu al-Maᶜarifī al-Osmania (Osmania Oriental Publications Bureau), Osmania University, 1952–74.

Renan, Ernest. *Les écrivains juifs français du XIVe siècle*. 1893. Reprint, Farnborough, England: Gregg, 1969.

Schacht, Joseph, and Max Meyerhof. "Maimonides against Galen, on Philosophy and Cosmogony." *Bulletin of the Faculty of Arts of the University of Egypt* 5, no. 1 (1937): 53–88 (Arabic section).

Schmucker, Werner. *Die pflanzliche und mineralische Materia medica im "Firdaus al-Ḥikma" des Ṭabarī*. Bonn: Selbstverlag des Orientalischen Seminars der Universität Bonn, 1969.

Schwartz, Dov. "Magiyah, maddaᶜ nisyoni u-metodah maddaᶜit be-mishnat ha-RaMBaM: Gishah u-parshanutah bime ha-benaim [Magic, experimental science, and scientific method in Maimonides' teachings]." In *Me-Romi l-Yirushalaim: Sefer Zikkaron le-Yoseph-Barukh Sermoneta* [Joseph Baruch sermoneta memorial volume], edited by Aviezer Ravitsky, 25–45 (English abstract: vii–viii). Jerusalem: The Hebrew University, 1998.

Sirat, Colette. "Une liste de manuscrits: Préliminaire à une nouvelle édition du *Dalālat al-Ḥāyryn.*" *Maimonidean Studies* 4 (2000): 109–33.

Soranus. *Sorani Gynaeciorum Libri IV. De signis Fracturarum. De fasciis. Vita Hippocratis secundum Soranum.* Edited by Johannes Ilberg. CMG 4. Leipzig: Teubner, 1927.

———. *Soranus' Gynecology.* Translated by Owsei Temkin, with the assistance of N. J. Eastman, L. Edelstein, and A. F. Guttmacher. Baltimore: Johns Hopkins University Press, 1956.

Steinschneider, Moritz. *Die arabischen Übersetzungen aus dem Griechischen.* 1889–96. Reprint, Graz, Austria: Akademische Druck- und Verlagsanstalt, 1960.

———. "Die griechischen Ärzte in arabischen Übersetzungen." *Virchows Archiv* 124 (1891): 115–36, 268–96, 455–87.

———. *Die hebräischen Handschriften der K. Hof- und Staatsbibliothek in München.* 2nd ed. Munich: Commission der Palm'schen Hofbuchhandlung, 1895.

———. *Die hebräischen Übersetzungen des Mittelalters und die Juden als Dolmetscher.* 1893. Reprint, Graz, Austria: Akademische Druck- und Verlagsanstalt, 1956.

———. *Verzeichniss der hebräischen Handschriften in Berlin.* 2 vols. 1878–97. Reprint in 1 vol., Hildesheim, Germany: Olms, 1980.

Strohmaier, G. "Der syrische und der arabische Galen." *Aufstieg und Niedergang der römischen Welt.* Part 2, vol. 37.2. Berlin: de Gruyter, 1994.

Ullmann, Manfred. *Die Medizin im Islam.* Leiden: Brill, 1970.

———. *Wörterbuch zu den griechisch-arabischen Übersetzungen des 9. Jahrhunderts.* Wiesbaden: Harrassowitz, 2002.

———. *Wörterbuch zu den griechisch-arabischen Übersetzungen des 9. Jahrhunderts: Supplement.* 2 vols. Wiesbaden: Harassowitz, 2006–7.

———. "Zwei spätantike Kommentare zu der hippokratischen Schrift *De morbis muliebribus.*" *Medizinhistorisches Journal* 12 (1977): 245–62.

Vajda, Georges. *Index général des manuscrits arabes musulmans de la Bibliothèque nationale de Paris.* Paris: Éditions du Centre national de la recherche scientifique, 1953.

Vogelstein, Hermann, and Paul Rieger. *Geschichte der Juden in Rom.* 2 vols. Berlin: Mayer und Müller, 1895–96.

Voorhoeve, Petrus, comp. *Handlist of Arabic Manuscripts in the Library of the University of Leiden and Other Collections in the Netherlands.* 2nd ed. The Hague: Leiden University Press, 1980.

Wörterbuch der klassischen arabischen Sprache. Edited by Deutsche Morgenländische Gesellschaft et al. Wiesbaden: Harrassowitz, 1957–.

Zahalon, Jacob. *Shemirat ha-beriʾut leha-RaMBaM: Perusho shel R. Yaʿakov Tsahalon ha-rofe le-hilkhot deʿot pereḳ dalet be-tosefet mavo ḳatsar le-ḥibbur "otsar ha-ḥayyim."* Edited by Zohar Amar. Jerusalem: Neveh-Tsuf, 2001.

Zonta, Mauro. "A Hebrew Translation of Hippocrates' *De superfoetatione:* Historical Introduction and Critical Introduction." *Aleph: Historical Studies in Science and Judaism* 3 (2003): 97–143.

Zotenberg, Hermann, ed. *Manuscrits orientaux: Catalogues des manuscrits hébreux et samaritains de la Bibliothèque impériale.* Paris: Imprimerie impériale, 1866.

Subject Index to the English Translation

bad, 111
bodily, 9, 57, 119
bodily, and sexual intercourse, 21
dominance of, in green bile, 133
in sharp substances, 119
phlegmatic, 11
salty substances dry, 117
sharp, 99
superfluous, 137
thick, 95
weak vision arises from, 91
morning, 25, 29, 65
motion of the soul, 37
mouth, 91, 99, 103
mūmiyā, 129
muscles, 7, 13, 89
musk, 125, 137

nature
activity of, 31
and dependence on laxatives, 33
balanced, of breasts, 15
human, relating to eating meat, 67
of a child and theriac, 35
of a person, 27
of animals close to that of humans, 99
of food, 63, 65
of liver, 81
of male body versus female body, 5
of often-used drugs, 121
of patient expands in temperate
bathwater, 57
of quails and sparrows, 87
of sour grapes, 89
Nature, 5, 13
nausea, 55, 91, 101
nazf, 5
neck, 3
nerves, 7, 13, 33, 73, 89
nose, 89
nosebleed, 31, 47, 55
nourishment, 25, 27, 67, 69, 85, 87, 115
nutriments, 95
nutrition, 69, 77
nuts. *See in* Botanicals Index

obstetric chair, 13
obstruction
of liver, 49, 59, 91
of liver and spleen, 103, 109
of spleen, 111
of uterus, 3

oil
astringent, 33
cooling, 23
good rubbing with, 41
in fomentations, embrocations, and
poultices, 119, 135–37
used for massage and rubbing, 23, 29, 43,
57, 115
with fruit, 109
See also oils, *in* Botanicals Index
old age, 31, 45. *See also* elderly; people, old
olive oil. *See* oils, *in* Botanicals Index
opthalmia, 51
organs
general, 21, 45, 61, 63, 97
lying on spinal column, 7
of childbirth, 3, 15
of the voice, 51
reproductive, 5
vital or major, 49, 59
os uteri, 13
oven, 67, 83
overfilling, 17, 41, 85, 93. *See also* satiation

palate, 103
partridges, 81–83, 87
passages, opening of, 23, 75, 93, 95, 111,
117. *See also* vessels; vein; channels
penis, 5
people, old, 23, 41, 137. *See also* elderly;
old age
people, young, 31, 35. *See also* children
perspiration, 97. *See also* sweat, sweating
pheasant, 81
phlegm, 39, 55, 93, 109
picra, 33
pigeons, 81, 87
pigs, milk of, 99. *See also* pork; swine, bile of
pitch, 133
placenta, 9, 11
plague, 115. *See also* epidemic diseases
plague spots, bloody, 93
plants, 25, 79
pleurisy, 53, 91, 101, 105
pneumonia, 53, 101
poison, 65, 79, 109, 111, 113–15, 137
poisoning, 79
pores, 57, 119, 135
pork, 67, 85. *See also* pigs, milk of; swine, bile of
potion, 105
potion of angels, 137
poultice, 51, 119, 135–37

Botanicals Index

absinthe wormwood, 33, 101, 111, 123
acorns, 83, 125
agaric, 109, 123
agrimony, 107, 111, 123
almonds, 79, 89, 123
almonds, bitter, 101
almonds, earth, 131
aloe, 33, 107, 111, 125
aloeswood, 125
amaranth, purple, 77, 91, 127
amber, yellow, 129
aneth. *See* dill
anise, 93, 129
apples, 79, 89, 125, 137
apricots, 83, 127
areca nut, 131
artichoke, 129
asafetida, 129
asarabacca, 121, 129
ash tree, fruit of 127
asparagus, 93, 121, 123
azarole, 125

balsam of Mecca, 125
bamboo, 175n177
bananas, 93, 123
barberry, 127
barley
  as drug, 125
  bread, 99
  groats, 27, 33, 81, 99
  gruel, 15, 81, 97, 99, 101, 105, 119
  juice, 85
  meal, 137
  sawīq, made with, 99, 135
basil, 79, 125
basil, bush, 123
bay laurel, 129

bdellium, 111, 119, 129
beans, broad, 119, 125
beans, mung, 125
beet, 67, 125
beet, wild, 125
behen, 127
ben oil tree, seed of, 129
bindweed, 171n121
bindweed, lesser, 33
birthwort, 125
bishop's weed, 79, 129
bitter ginger, 125
blackberry, 79, 107, 121, 125
black-eyed peas, 123
borage, 123
boxthorn, 127
bramble. *See* blackberry
buckthorns, 174n156

cabbage, 79, 83, 91, 107, 123
calamint, 160n90
calamint, lesser, 79, 129
caltrop, 125
camphor, 131
caper roots, skins of, 111
capers, 49, 109, 111, 129
caper spurge, 131
caraway, 129
caraway, wild, 129
cardamom, 123
carob, 125
carrot, 121, 125
carrot, seed of wild, 121, 129
cassia, 111, 129, 137
cauliflower, 123
celandine, 129
celery, 29, 79, 121, 129
celery, seed of mountain, 79

chestnut, 79
nutmeg, 171n118
pomegranate, 173n152
sandarac, 123
terebinth, 33, 111, 119, 125
truffles, 83, 127
turmeric, 129
turnips, 77, 87, 93, 125
turpeth, 129

valerian, 121
valerian, Indian, 113
vetch, bitter, 119, 123

vine, 107
violets, 125

walnuts, 79, 81, 89, 109, 127
watermelon, 67, 79, 81, 83, 127
waybread, 127
wheat, 75, 81, 83, 119, 123, 135
willow, 125
wormwood, 129
wormwood, absinthe, 33, 101, 111, 123

zarnab, 129

Addenda and Corrigenda
to *Medical Aphorisms*
Volumes 1–15

Medical Aphorisms: Treatises 1–5

Arabic text:

1.31 (p. 14, line 14): تعيا .Read: تعبا

English translation:

3.15 (p. 37, line 11); 3.20 (p. 38, line 6); 3.30 (p. 40, lines 19–20): "main organs" (Ar. الأعضاء الأصلية). Read "elementary parts" (i.e., the homogeneous [homoeomerous] parts, such as arteries, veins, nerves, bones, cartilages, membranes, ligaments, and the various coats)

3.72 (p. 51, lines 25–26): "(namely, the other things which change its temperament)" Read: "(namely, the other things which change its temperament or dissolve its continuity)"

Medical Aphorisms: Treatises 6–9

Arabic text:

6.10 (p. 3, line 11): يعتد به .Read: يعتدّ به

6.13 (p. 4, line 5): الرمص .Read: الرمض

7.63 (p. 39, line 10): أربغة .Read: أربعة

7.65 (p. 39 line 15): أذا .Read: إذا

7.73 (p. 41, line 16): تمثل .Read: تمثّل

8.17 (p. 46, line 2): تجذب الفضول نحو. Read: تجذب الفضول التي مالت نحو

9.11 (p. 61, line 14): على أصل. Read: على أصل اللسان

9.113 (p. 83, line 13): يغتة. Read: بغتة

English translation:

6.10 (p. 3, lines 20–21): "and neither pain nor fever develops." Read: "and no considerable pain nor fever develops"

6.29 (p. 15, line 29); 7.11 (p. 26, line 15); 8.14 (p. 45, line 12); 8.58 (p. 54, line 12): "main organs" (Ar. الأعضاء الأصلية). Read "elementary parts" (i.e., the homogeneous [homoeomerous] parts, such as arteries, veins, nerves, bones, cartilages, membranes, ligaments, and the various coats)

8.17 (p. 46, lines 3–4): "attract the superfluities towards." Read: "attract the superfluities that tend towards"

9.11 (p. 61, line 25): "[of the tongue]." Read: "of the tongue"

9.79 (p. 76, line 13): "and the soul becomes upset." Add footnote to "the soul": I.e., the stomach, cf. aphorisms 9.51, 55.

9.108 (p. 82, line 23): "marshmallow." Read: "mallow"

Medical Aphorisms: Treatises 10–15

Arabic text:

12.24 (p. 34, line 6): لألطف. Read: بألطف

13.36 (p. 47, line 16): يغري. Read: يغرّي

13.38 (p. 48, line 3): استفراغه أوّل. Read: استفراغ هؤلاء

13.43 (p. 48, line 16): ومغرّية. Read: ومغرية

13.52 (p. 51, line 5): يغري. Read: يغرّي

15.19 (p. 60, line 8): المحلوق. Read: المخلوق

15.22 (p. 61, line 1): مضرّة. Read: مضرّة من وجه آخر

15.70 (p. 71, line 3): ثلاثة أصابع. Read: ثلاثة أصابع أو أربع

English translation:

10.61 (p. 16, line 16): "main organs" (Ar. الأعضاء الأصلية). Read "elementary parts" (i.e., the homogeneous [homoeomerous] parts, such as arteries, veins, nerves, bones, cartilages, membranes, ligaments, and the various coats)

13.38 (p. 48, line 5): "Such a person should be, first of all, evacuated." Read: "Such a person should be evacuated"

15.15 (p. 59, line 13): "a site that has tendons and nerves." Read: "a site that has tendons and nerves or veins"

15.22 (p. 61, line 2): "will not come to any harm because of that." Read: "will not come to any harm in another aspect because of that"

15.41: (p. 64, lines 26–27): "We are forced to cauterize if the hemorrhage is caused by corrosion or putrefaction affecting it." Read: "We are forced to cauterize if the hemorrhage is caused by corrosion or putrefaction affecting the organ"

15.70 (p. 71, lines 4–5): "three thumbs." Read: "three or four thumbs"

GERRIT BOS was born in the Netherlands and educated there and in Jerusalem and London. He is proficient in classical and Semitic languages, as well as in Jewish and Islamic studies. He has been a research assistant at the Free University in Amsterdam, a research fellow and lecturer at University College in London, a tutor in Jewish studies at Leo Baeck College in London, a Wellcome Institute research fellow, and chair of the Martin Buber Institute of Jewish Studies at the University of Cologne. He currently resides in the Netherlands with his wife and three children.

Professor Bos is widely published in the fields of Jewish studies, Islamic studies, Judeo-Arabic texts, and medieval Islamic science and medicine, having many books and articles to his credit. In addition to preparing the Medical Works of Moses Maimonides, Professor Bos is also involved with a series of medical-botanical Arabic-Hebrew-Romance synonym texts written in Hebrew characters, an edition of Ibn al-Jazzār's *Zād al-musāfir* (Viaticum), and an edition of Marwān Ibn Janāḥ, *Kitāb al-Talkhīṣ*. He is a Member of Honor of the Argentinean Society for the History of Medicine.